A Patient's Perspective on Spastic Tetraparesis Diagnosis:

Specially Abled

A Patient's Perspective on Spastic Tetraparesis Diagnosis:

Specially Abled

By

Bianca Wiersema and Dragoș Sardaru

Cambridge
Scholars
Publishing

A Patient's Perspective on Spastic Tetraparesis Diagnosis: Specially Abled

By Bianca Wiersema and Dragoș Sardaru

This book first published 2024

Cambridge Scholars Publishing

Lady Stephenson Library, Newcastle upon Tyne, NE6 2PA, UK

British Library Cataloguing in Publication Data
A catalogue record for this book is available from the British Library

ISBN (10): 1-5275-5306-X
ISBN (13): 978-1-5275-5306-4

I dedicate this book to the person that turned impossible into possible: My mum.

Every day is a new opportunity to live

CONTENTS

LIST OF TABLES

FOREWORD

I hope that this book will be of great use to you. The idea of writing it arose in my mind as I encountered many difficulties and had so many unanswered questions about what the diagnosis of spastic tetraparesis implies. Beyond the physical limitations, which cannot be cured, its purpose is to show you that you can get good results if you work hard. This book aims to provide a broader look at the challenges that a diagnosis of spastic tetraparesis can bring, as well as a perspective on the creativity and flexibility required to overcome the obstacles that arise when facing such a diagnosis.

I would like to begin by thanking my family for all their help throughout this ordeal; even when I thought there was no hope, they never gave up and showed me that everything I really needed was right in front of my eyes. I just had to grab it.

I would also like to thank those who told me I could not do it and that I would not make it, because it was through them that I met the right people who showed and proved to me that I CAN AND WILL MAKE IT THROUGH, but only with great effort. Thus, our satisfaction and successes were commensurate with our efforts, and we learned that in life you have to climb, in order to enjoy the beautiful view of how far you have come. You should learn to enjoy the journey rather than the destination.

When speaking about a person with different abilities, it would be better to say: "Person X is diagnosed with Y diagnosis." If you replace "is diagnosed" with "person X HAS Y diagnosis" you imply that the person and the diagnosis are one and the same and that Y is a part of the person's identity, which it is not. Apart from the medical diagnosis, a person is a human being with emotions, experiences, personality, and attitudes. The fact that a person has been diagnosed with a medical or psychological condition only tells you what kind of limitations this person may have, not who or what the person is, and what kind of extraordinary abilities he has or is still developing. What a person chooses to be – his passions, his fears, and his successes – are not conditioned, determined, or resulted from the person's diagnosis. So, address the person by his name.

Although there may not appear to be a significant difference between the two phrases at first glance, to reduce a person's value to a diagnosis — obtained as a result of medical evaluations—is like putting a human being in a cage with chains: the person will feel useless, small, insignificant, powerless, without any perspective.

On the other hand, if you see through, the person who uses such phrases — when referring to someone with different abilities —is actually the one who is chained by one's own thoughts, because instead of seeing possibilities, they see defeats and limitations.

I hope that this book will take you on a journey where you discover the person rather than the diagnosis. It gives you answers to questions that seem unanswered, the courage to face your demons and make your journey easier, and last but not least it gives you the tools to enjoy life as much as possible. Because each person's manifestations are unique, the information provided here should not be generalized.

What Dr. Cîrstoveanu Cătălin said best describes what I want this book to mean, and I quote: "Miracles happen, but they go hand in hand with a lot of work." (Cîrstoveanu 2020).

ACKNOWLEDGMENTS

First and foremost, I would like to express my gratitude to my brother, Theodor-Constantin Wiersema, and to my special father Hisko, who raised me, showed me the world—as I could not go on my own to see the world, —taught me patience, gave me hope, and reminded me over and over again that "the strongest you are between your ears" meaning that the strongest you are in your mind the better you can cope with life. He was the one who realized I was deaf! He taught me how to swim, and carried me all over in his arms and on his back. He would get up every night to cover me and check on me to see if I was okay. Last but not least I am grateful to my mother, who has been by my side since the first second of my life and has tried to find solutions where she was told they did not exist.

Taking their feedback into account, I attempted to make this book as accessible as possible.

In addition, I would like to express my gratitude to Cătălin Andrei Cibotaru for all the explanations given in connection with this diagnosis, as well as for his patience in explaining everything in a simple way, allowing for the transfer of knowledge in this book.

I would also like to thank Marijn Peters and Brigitte Ioniță for their valuable feedback on the book's content. Claudia-Andreea Păduraru has the copyright of all the adapted illustrations/graphic designs and Iuliana-Ilinca Vieriu owns the copyright of the pictures[1] (unless otherwise specified).

I express my gratitude to Cambridge Scholars Publishing for their enthusiastic response to this book's initiative and for their assistance in its printing.

Finally, I would like to thank everyone I met during my studying years. Although the road was difficult and challenging, testing all of my limits from each and every perspective, the variety of people I met provided me with the opportunity to learn about different perspectives on this diagnosis,

[1] If you would like to use the pictures, graphic designs, or illustrations in any other context, you will need to get a written request from Bianca Wiersema and the copyright owner.

which greatly aided me in writing this book and they proved to me that in life I have to appreciate the little things because they are the ones that change our lives: the smiles I bring, the kisses and hugs I give… they may seem so little and yet they mean so much.

I changed lives by moving people's souls.

I would be happy if I could make your life better by making the diagnosis more understandable.

CHAPTER 1

A MATTER OF SECONDS

I was born at 6 and a half months; I weighed a kilogram and I had hypoxia. The doctors said I would not survive, due to my premature birth, and I had no Apgar score. I only started breathing a few minutes after I was born, due to the doctors' intervention. Doctor Stamatin saved my life that night...

In other words, I failed from the start by not being born at the proper time. Who would have said that despite my failure I would still be among the first in class during school?

My premature birth did not come alone, it came hand in hand with an incurable diagnosis. And the icing on the cake is that I have the most serious form of cerebral palsy, which occurs in 5% of cases: spastic tetraparesis. In addition, I had strabismus at birth — which I corrected — and deafness – corrected with hearing aids – the whole caboodle.

After I stayed in hospital for the first 3 months, at 6 months I started physiotherapy, under the guidance of Doctor Stamatin who realized that something was wrong and that is how my journey began: physiotherapy, speech therapy, eye muscle exercises...I had a serious job until I was 10 years old 😊.

At a year and a half, I went to a neurologist, the late Doctor Popescu, the only person who told my mother that I would do well intellectually but I would never run, and that my life would depend on physical therapy without which I would not be able to live. That was the hope and confirmation that things in my life would enter a so-called "normal" phase.

I tried everything from massage to electrostimulation and balneo-physiotherapy. Unfortunately, many physiotherapists focused on increasing my muscle strength, which aggravated my spasticity while others focused on the things I could not do, even after trying those things for a long time, instead of focusing on what I could do. The massage was ineffective, and I changed over 20 physiotherapists in my lifetime. What can I say, I like variety!

I underwent three tendon lengthening operations. After two surgeries I was not allowed to stand on my feet for 3 months. As a result, the recovery was very long and painful.

Regression was inevitable and I honestly admit that there were times in my life when frustration and fatigue peaked, but my mother brought a special person into my life—I call him "The Best of the Best!" —a physiotherapist who focused on what I can do and for the first time in 16 years, I felt that doing physiotherapy is not meant to be only pain.

When the time came to start school, I was denied admission to public nursery schools, so I attended a private nursery supported by a Dutch foundation. I was later turned down by a state school, so my parents enrolled me in a private school where I met my first teacher who decided to believe in me. I thank her for everything she has taught me.

Unfortunately, 2 years later I moved to a state school and for years I had to go up 2 floors to my class until the 10th grade when, to my relief, the headmistress, who understood that the effort I was making was superhuman, moved my class to the ground floor. I thank her from the bottom of my heart and for being the kind, caring, sensitive soul I so desperately needed in my life!

Sadly, my classmates were not friendly, I was always sitting alone at my desk, but the good part was that I could spread my notebooks on the whole desk, and no one copied from me (what can I say, I was one of the best at school, even if I did not become the head of promotion).

Mathematics was not my strong point, but luckily my mother found the teacher who made me understand the secrets of mathematics. An exceptional teacher, who, for 4 years, visited every weekend, voluntarily, to teach me mathematical logic. I am deeply grateful to her for her unusual methods and her patience with me! Her friend, an English teacher, taught me to spice English up with a little salt and pepper! And it tasted really wonderful! Remembering historical facts was also a challenge for me, but luckily, I met the person who captivated me with his skills in telling historical events, which helped me memorize battles and many other facts, making learning history fun!

Time flies, college is coming! I wanted to study psychology, and was not I happy when I entered Alexandru Ioan Cuza University in Iași with a scholarship! But the rector decided that it is better to study at a distance because they will not make the place accessible and that there is no point in trying, because, anyway, I will not finish, that is what he foresaw.

I was on the brink of having a breakdown. But when someone closes a door, a window opens. That open window was The Netherlands, where I studied psychology.

The irony of life made me fall in love with neurology...and all led to the completion of a master's degree in neuropsychology. Being the first in Romania with a master's degree in this specialization, they just have to recognize it in my country! But what can I say, it is harder when you are first, but I certainly will not be the last. And I certainly will not give up! I am a fighter, still!

So much about me, let's see what spastic tetraparesis means!

CHAPTER 2

IN FACT, WHAT IS SPASTIC TETRAPARESIS? DEFINITIONS OF INTRODUCTORY TERMS, PLEGIA VERSUS PARESIS, AND CEREBRAL PALSY CLASSIFICATIONS

When William J. Little (1862) linked certain deformities to "abnormal parturition, difficult labors, premature birth, and asphyxia neonatorum," he made a brilliant contribution to clinical medicine. Nelson and Ellenberg (1978) described the disorder formerly known as Little's disease, now known as cerebral palsy (CP), as "not a single disease, but rather a group of conditions differing in topographic distribution, specific manifestations, and associated handicaps, and probably (but to a degree as yet unknown) varying in etiology." Cohen and Kohn (1979) characterized cerebral palsy as a syndrome rather than a clear-cut diagnosis, and Minear (1956) highlights that cerebral palsy treatment should focus on symptoms rather than etiology.

Cerebral palsy is thought to be caused by a central nervous system lesion that produces motor dysfunction as well as sensory, cognitive, and emotional abnormalities in many cases. The lesion is non-progressive and is acquired early in life, though it can occur during the neonatal, perinatal, or postnatal periods. The present emphasis on developmental disorders, such as cerebral palsy, should assist to bolster the latter requirement, namely that the handicap is acquired early enough in the maturational process to impact normal advancement through developmental milestones (Lindeman 1981).

Cerebral palsy affects 1.5-2.5 out of every 1,000 newborns worldwide; developing countries having a higher prevalence. Cerebral palsy is a heterogeneous group of "movement and posture disorders" of varying types and severity caused by an injury or a non-progressive defect of the immature brain in full development, the etiological agent acting in the antenatal/perinatal and postnatal period until the age of approximately 3-5 years. In 20% of cases, the origin of cerebral palsy is unknown (Diaconu 2008, 247).

The ability to generate sufficient tension in a muscle for the purposes of posture and movement is defined as strength (Smidt and Rogers, 1982). Strength is a result of both the musculoskeletal properties of the muscle and its neural activation. The inability to generate normal levels of force is defined as weakness. The severity of weakness in a patient with a cerebral cortex lesion can range from total or severe loss of muscle activity, known as "plegia", to mild or partial loss of muscle activity, known as "paresis." (Shumway-Cook and H.Woollacott, 2011, chap. 5).

Paralysis is defined as the presence of a motor deficit and is classified into two types: paresis and plegia.

Paresis is defined as a decrease in voluntary motor unit recruitment and represents an inability or difficulty in recruiting skeletal motor units to generate torque or movement. This causes an inability to recruit and/or modulate motor neurons, resulting in a loss of movement. Paresis, or weakness, is a primary neuromuscular impairment that affects the number, type, and frequency of discharge of motor neurons required for force production during gait (Duncan and Badke, 1987). Paresis is characterized by weakness or partial loss of voluntary muscle movement, as well as impaired movement, implying a partial motor deficit, but the upper or/and lower limbs still respond to sensory or motor stimuli (Davis, 2019; Piseru and Piseru, 2023.). Plegia is defined as the complete inability to perform voluntary movements. Plegia is a type of paralysis characterized by the loss of muscle control over one or more muscles. If there is sensory as well as motor damage, paralysis may be followed by a loss of sensation (sensory loss) in the affected area, implying total loss of voluntary movement. Plainly said, paralysis is the inability to move, sense touch, or control bodily sensations as a result of an accident or medical condition. However, paralysis can take various forms and affects people differently. The distinction between plegia and paresis will guide the establishment of an appropriate prognosis and recovery program, involving various means and strategies of the therapy plan. Paresis implies the development of pre-existing motor control, whereas plegia implies the initiation of voluntary motor control (Piseru and Piseru, 2023).

According to Lindemann (1981, chap. 5), cerebral palsy types are classified based on motor symptom complexes and topography (the parts of the body involved). To appreciate motor function, the reader is invited to extend his arm straight out in front of him, palm up, and bend it. The muscles inside the arm (flexors) contract while the muscles outside the arm (extensors) relax. Signals from the brain via the spinal cord cause these opposing muscles to move in perfect coordination. The movement is monitored and modified simultaneously based on sensory feedback from the muscles. Certain primitive and automatic reflexes are also used by the body to keep functions like balance and body coordination in an upright position. Cerebral palsy is defined as a disruption in the system that signals this finely tuned motor functioning. According to Johnston (1976), this is due to an inappropriate balance of voluntary and involuntary controls, stimulating and suppressing influences, and flexion and extensor postures.

Spasticity is a term used to describe a disturbance characterized by a hyperactive muscle stretch reflex. Muscles will be tight (hypertonic), and movement will be jerky, due to the sudden relaxation of hypertonic muscles and spasms of contraction and relaxation. Athetosis (Fig. 2-1) occurs when a disturbance is characterized by an abnormal amount of involuntary motion, resulting in bizarre, purposeless, writhing movements. Ataxia is a disorder characterized primarily by incoordination and poor balance. Other less common classifications of motor function include rigidity, tremor, and atonia (Lindemann, 1981, chap. 5).

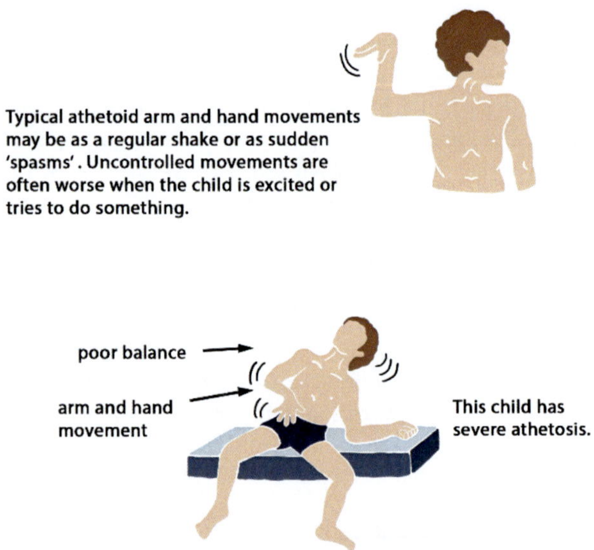

Fig. 2-1. This picture shows a child who has severe athetosis (adapted from Werner, 1987, chap. 9)

Cerebral palsy manifests itself differently depending on which part of the brain is damaged, and the nature of the damage (Kolb and Whishaw, 2015, chap. 24). The causes of cerebral palsy vary and are classified into four major categories based on the nature of the damage, as shown in Table 2-1.

Table 2-1. Potential Causes of Cerebral Palsy

Hereditary

Static—familial athetosis, familial paraplegia, familial tremor

Progressive—demyelinating diseases of viral or undetermined origin (chromosomal breakages are rare in cerebral palsy, as are disorders of metabolism)

Congenital (acquired in utero)

Infectious rubella, toxoplasmosis, cytomegalic inclusions, herpes simplex, other viral or infectious agents

Maternal anoxia, carbon monoxide poisoning, strangulation, anemia, hypotension associated with spinal anesthesia, placental infarcts, placenta abruptio

Prenatal cerebral hemorrhage, maternal toxemia, direct trauma, maternal bleeding, diathesis

Prenatal anoxia, twisting or kinking of the cord

Miscellaneous toxins, drugs

Perinatal (obstetrical)

Mechanical anoxia—respiratory obstruction, narcotism due to oversedation with drugs, placenta previa or abruptio, hypotension associated with spinal anesthesia, breech delivery with delay of the after-coming head

Trauma—hemorrhage associated with dystocia, disproportions and malpositions of labor, sudden pressure changes, precipitate delivery, caesarean delivery

Complications of birth—"small for date" babies, prematurity, immaturity, dysmaturity, postmaturity, hyperbilirubinemia and isoimmunization factors (kernicterus due to Rh factor, ABO incompatibility), hemolytic disorders, respiratory distress disorders, syphilis, meningitis, and other infections, drug-addiction reactions, hypoglycemic reactions, hypocalcemic reactions

Postnatal–Infancy

Trauma—subdural hematoma, skull fracture, cerebral contusion

Infections—meningitis, encephalitis, brain abscess

Vascular accidents—congenital cerebral aneurism, thrombosis, embolism, hypertensive encephalopathy, sudden pressure changes

Toxins—lead, arsenic, coal-tar derivatives

Anoxia—carbon monoxide poisoning, strangulation, high-altitude and deep-pressure anoxia, hypoglycemia

Neoplastic and late neurodevelopmental defects—tumor, cyst, progressive hydrocephalus

Eric Denhoff, "Medical Aspects," in Cerebral Palsy: A Developmental Disability, ed. William M. Cruickshank, 3rd rev. ed. (Syracuse: Syracuse University Press, 1976), 35. © Syracuse University Press. Reproduced with permission from the publisher.

Clinically, the following types of cerebral palsy have been identified (Diaconu 2008, 247-252):

1. pyramidal or spastic
2. extrapyramidal or dystonic-dyskinetic
3. CP- ataxic form
4. CP- atonal form
5. CP- mixed form

Spastic types of CP are the most common, with increased hypertension until contracture as a manifestation, which is generally major on the flexor muscles at the upper limbs (UL) and on the extensor muscles at the lower limbs (LL), and always predominant on the distal segments.

The following clinical presentations can be distinguished based on the severity and topographic distribution of the paralysis (Fig.2-2):

- Hemiplegia is a motor injury to a hemibody.
- Diplegia with bilateral spasticity affects both sides of the body, primarily the LL but also the UL.
- Tetraplegia affects all four limbs, but the UL is often more severely affected than the LL.

The incidence of cerebral palsy is presented in Table 2-2.

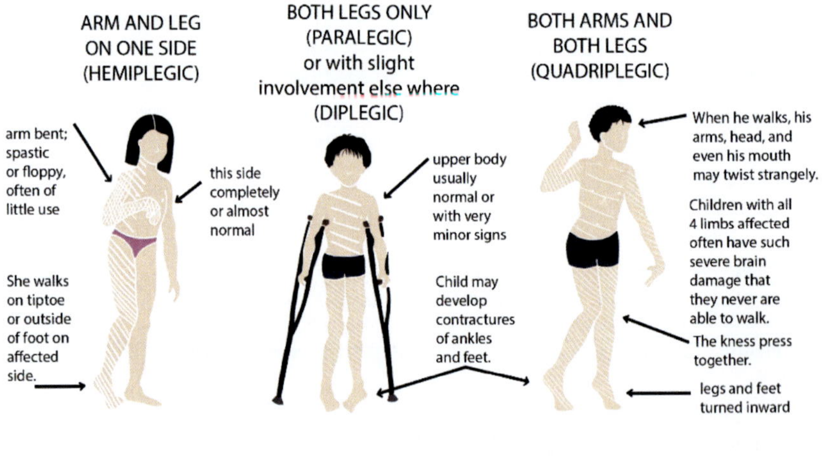

Figure 2-2. Hemiplegia, diplegia and quadriplegia (adapted from Werner, 1987, chap. 9).

Table 2-2: Cerebral Palsy Types with Prevalence

CEREBRAL PALSY	
Spastic hemiplegia	25 to 40%
Spastic diplegia	10 to 33%
Spastic quadriplegia	9 to 43%
Extrapyramidal (including athetoid ataxic and dystonic forms)	9 to 22%
Mixed	9 to 22%

Adapted from Lindeman (1981), which was adapted from Nelson and Ellenberg (1978). The prevalence rate of cerebral palsy at 4.6 at 1,000 births, at 7 years of age. The study had 54.000 of children.

The Apgar score is used to assess an infant's readiness for life outside the womb. The Apgar score has five dimensions: color, heart rate, reflexes, muscle tone, and respiration. Each dimension receives a score of 0, 1, or 2. As a result, the Apgar score quantifies clinical signs of neonatal depression such as cyanosis or pallor, bradycardia, a low reflex response to stimulation, hypotonia, and apnea or gasping respiration (Apgar et al., 1958). It closely correlates with gestational age, according to Stamatin, Păduraru, and Avasiloaiei (2009), with premature newborns having a lower value, being evaluated at 1, 5, 10, and 20 minutes.

From birth to 12 months, there are several important signs of cerebral palsy (as shown in Fig. 2.3), but there are also delays in different phases of normal development when compared to a baby who does not have cerebral palsy. The normal development stages through which a healthy baby goes compared to one with spastic tetraparesis are shown in Fig. 2.4.

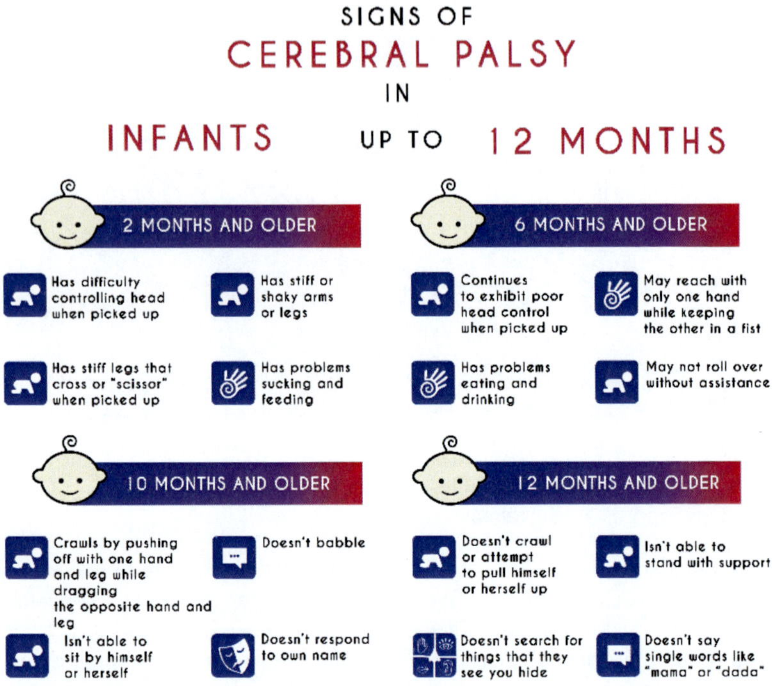
SIGNS OF
CEREBRAL PALSY
IN
INFANTS UP TO 12 MONTHS
2 MONTHS AND OLDER
Has difficulty controlling head when picked up
Has stiff or shaky arms or legs
Has stiff legs that cross or "scissor" when picked up
Has problems sucking and feeding
6 MONTHS AND OLDER
Continues to exhibit poor head control when picked up
May reach with only one hand while keeping the other in a fist
Has problems eating and drinking
May not roll over without assistance
10 MONTHS AND OLDER
Crawls by pushing off with one hand and leg while dragging the opposite hand and leg
Doesn't babble
Isn't able to sit by himself or herself
Doesn't respond to own name
12 MONTHS AND OLDER
Doesn't crawl or attempt to pull himself or herself up
Isn't able to stand with support
Doesn't search for things that they see you hide
Doesn't say single words like "mama" or "dada"

Fig. 2.3. This image shows signs of cerebral palsy in babies up from 2 months up to 1 year (adapted from NeuroGen Brain & Spine Institute, 2008).

Table 2-4. The drawings on the left depict how normal babies move at various developmental stages. The images in the middle and on the right depict how a baby with spastic tetraparesis might perform the same activity (adapted from Lesson 20: Disability and Rehabilitation Part 2 – WikiEducator, 2007).

Normal development	Spastic tetraparesis development	
	At 3 Months	
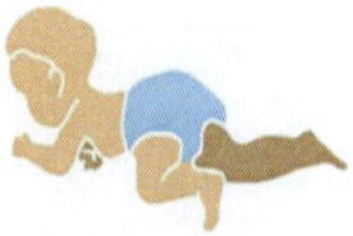	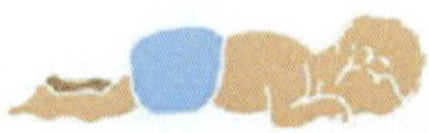	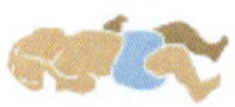
Lie straight on stomach	Lies flat on belly	Lies straight on back
Holds head up well	Cannot lift head	Push back head
Push up on arms	Cannot push up on arms	Two arms bent
Legs flexible	Still and stiff legs	Two legs bent
Brings hands together	Do not move the hands	Cannot bring hands together

At 6 Months			
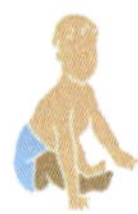	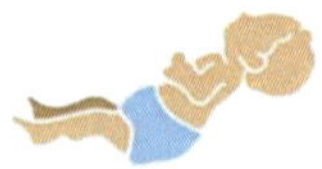	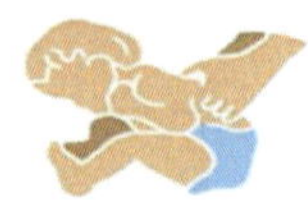	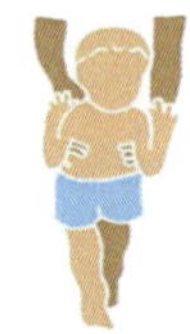
Sits leaning on his hands	Cannot sit	Stiff arms Fisted hands and cannot sustain on them	Arms pull back
Keeps head	Head falls back when sitting	Cannot keep head up	Head goes in front
Keeps back straight	Stiff back	Round back cannot keep straight Stiff muscles	Stiff back
Can take the weight by standing	Stiff legs	Stiff legs	Stiff legs crossed like scissors Tiptoe standing

At 9 Months		
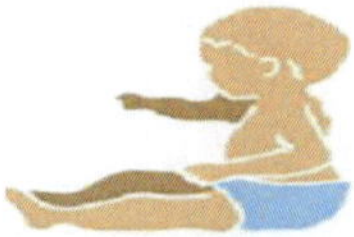	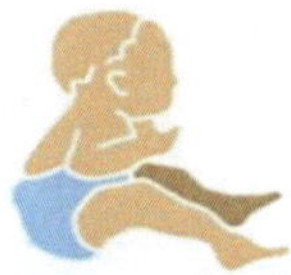	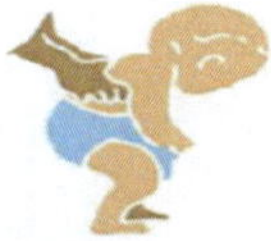
Sits alone	Sits with support in the back	Sits with support in the back
Reaches out	Round back	Cannot lift head good
Can use hands to play	Poor use of hands to play	Cannot use hands to play
Flexible legs	Stiff legs	Cannot keep the weight on his legs when standing
Can support himself	Pointed toes when put in standing	Cannot support himself

At 12 months		
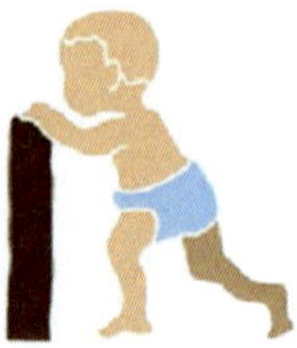	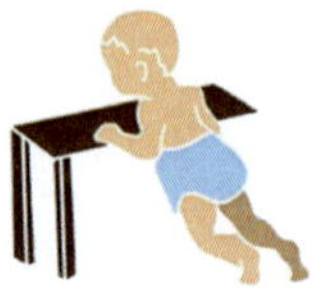	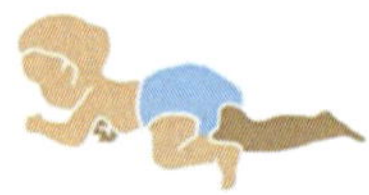
Crawls well	Difficulties pulling to stand	Cannot crawl
Pulls to stand	He pulls on his toes by holding something Pointed toes	Cannot stand by holding something
Can drag himself	Cannot drag himself	Cannot use any side of the body to drag himself

At 18 months		
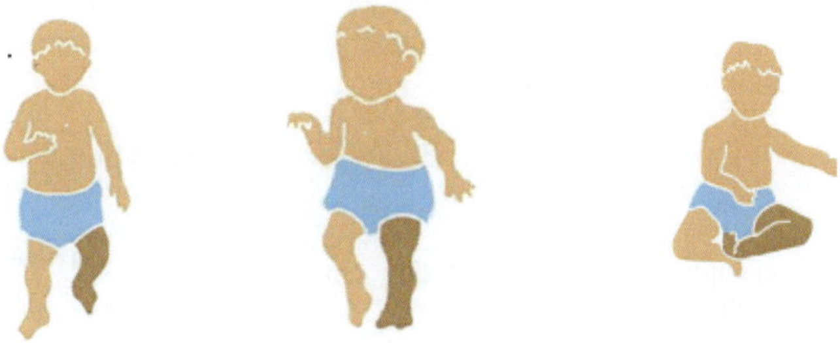		
Walks alone	Cannot walk alone	Cannot walk alone
Stands alone	Poor standing Poor balance	Cannot stand alone
Sits straight	Cannot sit straight	Cannot keep balance while sitting
Use both hands	Both arms are stiff	Cannot use both hands
Both legs flexible and keep weight when walking	Legs stiff Tiptoe walking on both legs	Legs stiff Cannot walk

Note: The brown color represents the left side of the body and the light brown represents the right side of the body.

Case study: Spastic tetraparesis(ST)

Spastic tetraparesis is the most severe form of CP, depicting in 5% of the cases and having its etiology in severe brain malformations, central nervous system(CNS) infections, genetic factors, prematurity, and perinatal complications. The clinical picture is characterized by the occurrence of spasticity and pyramidal syndrome (Diaconu, 2008, 251).

Spastic tetraparesis clinical features and dysfunctions in children (Diaconu, 2008, 251-252).

- In the supine position (with the face-up), as shown in Fig. 2.5, there is increased extensor spasticity: the head is hyperextended, the thorax and shoulders are retracted, and the LL are extended-adducted-intrarotated with plantar flexion of the foot. UL are abducted-extrarotated with closed fists and police in adduction. Hip dislocation can occur as a result of adductor contractions.

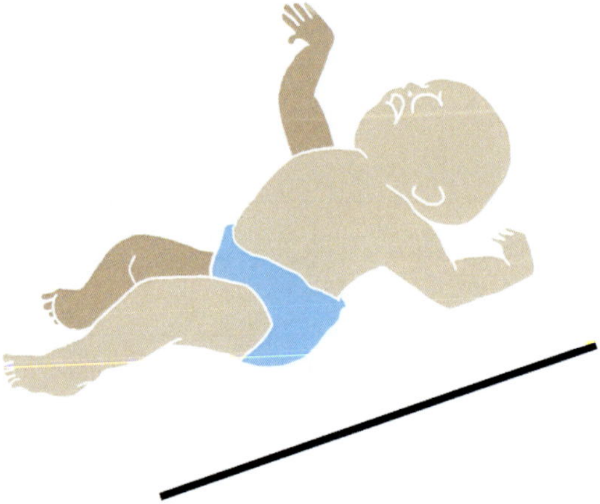

Fig. 2.5. In the supine position, the head, shoulder girdle, and arms are extended, and the legs are stretched out like a newborn (adapted from Hinchcliffe, 2007, chap. 3). Note: The brown color represents the left side of the body and the light brown represents the right side of the body.

- In the prone position (with the face-down), as shown in Fig. 2.6, there is global flexor synergy. The thorax is flexed, the arms are in adduction and flexed under the thorax, the LL are in flexion, and the infant is unable to rotate the head to clear the airways.

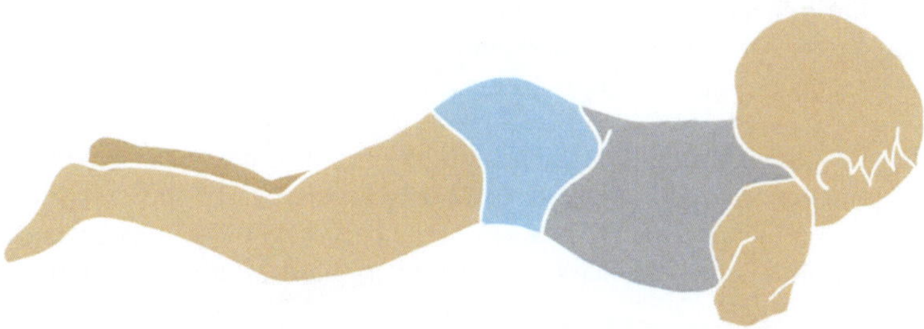

Fig. 2.6. In the prone position, flexion pattern (adapted from Hinchcliffe, 2007, chap. 3). Note: The brown color represents the left side of the body and the light brown represents the right side of the body.

- Walking on all four members is difficult because the semi-flexed UL are rigid, which is why they prefer to sit on their knees, sit, or crawl, which will exacerbate flexor spasticity and lead to thoracic and lower limb contractions and flexion deformities over time.

- The asymmetry of the thorax and the obliquity of the pelvis are determined by very pronounced asymmetric tonic neck reflexes (ATNR). The child is unable to lift his head or bend his hip, preventing him from sitting in a sitting position. Rolling is impossible due to shoulder retraction. The amount of spontaneous movement is reduced and done in blocks. Block movement occurs when the anterior and posterior hemibodies move in the same direction at the same time.

- Due to a lack of head control, other issues such as mastication and swallowing problems may occur in people with severe ST (damage to the cortico-bulbar pathways affects the muscles of the lower face which can lead to difficulties in mastication, swallowing, dysarthria, hypersalivation, hypomimia). Some people, especially at night, may experience severe breathing difficulties.

- In addition to microcephaly, language difficulties (lack of language or primitive dysarthric language), severe mental retardation, cranial nerve palsies, optic atrophy, and strabismus can occur. Furthermore, if orthopedic complications like hip dislocation, scoliosis, or leg deformity occur, more physiotherapy on the affected body part may be beneficial.

- Early neuromotor reeducation can help to prevent contractures and/or worsening of contractures, as well as improve functional prognosis, though motor progress is modest and slow.

- People with mild ST may be able to sit in a sitting position without assistance and then stand up if they receive early and consistent physiotherapy, but the chances of the person walking independently are slim due to balance issues and a very narrow base of support.

- Cognitively, a child with medium or mild TS because of a lack of handling, will have great difficulties with spatial orientation, a poor understanding of the body scheme, and thus a significant limitation of autonomy in daily life as well as in terms of performance. The handicap will be more severe in those suffering from mental retardation, language difficulties, visual impairment, or epilepsy.

- Problems related to this diagnosis can impair all aspects of life, including motor, speech, hearing, intellectual, emotional, and social functioning, as well as self-concept, and job adjustment (Lindemann, 1981, chap. 5).

These issues could be significantly made worse by following inadequate training and education.

Illustrations of a spastic position when lying on one's back and when sitting are shown in Figures 2.7, 2.8 and 2.9.

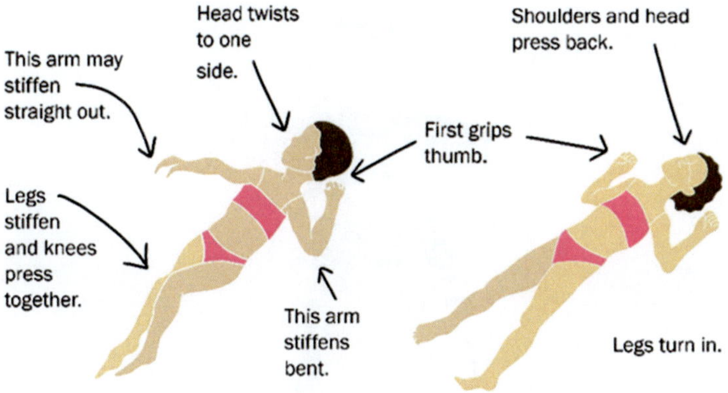

Fig. 2.7. A spastic position when lying on one's back (adapted from Werner, 1987, chap. 9). Note: The brown color represents the left side of the body and the light brown represents the right side of the body.

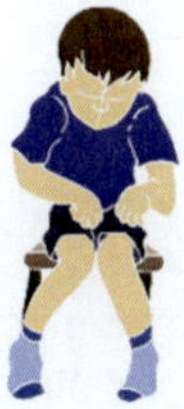

Fig. 2.8. Sitting with the head flexed and the arms in a flexion pattern (adapted from Hinchcliffe, 2007, chap. 3).

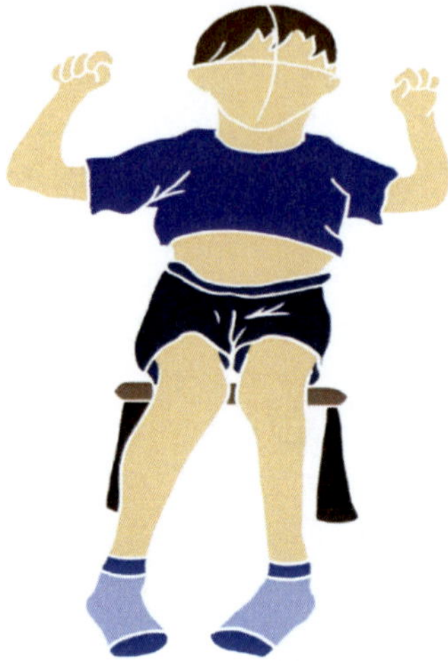

Fig. 2.9. In a sitting position with the head raised and the arms extended (adapted from Hinchcliffe, 2007, chap. 3).

If the child's head hangs back, do not pull him up in the manner shown in Fig. 2.10 on the right side. Check to see if his neck muscles tighten as you begin to lift him. If not, do not pull him up. Also, do not pull the child up in this manner if it causes his legs to straighten stiffly. If a child with cerebral palsy becomes stiff when his arms are pulled, try pulling him up by pulling his shoulder blades forward as shown in Fig. 2.10, on the left side. (Werner 1987, chap. 35).

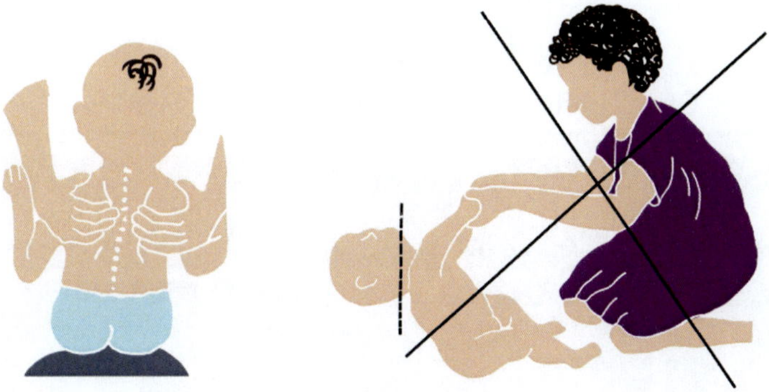

Fig. 2.10. How to grab the child correctly (adapted from Werner, 1987, chap. 35)

The Gross Motor Function Classification System (GMFCS) is a multi-level categorization technique that aids in illustrating varying levels of severity in people with cerebral palsy. The GMFCS is divided into five levels, with lower levels corresponding to milder forms of CP and higher levels indicating increased severity. All forms and severity levels of cerebral palsy can be described using the Gross Motor Function Classification System. It takes into account a person's voluntary motions, age, and functional abilities in a range of situations (Reiter and Walsh, n.d.).

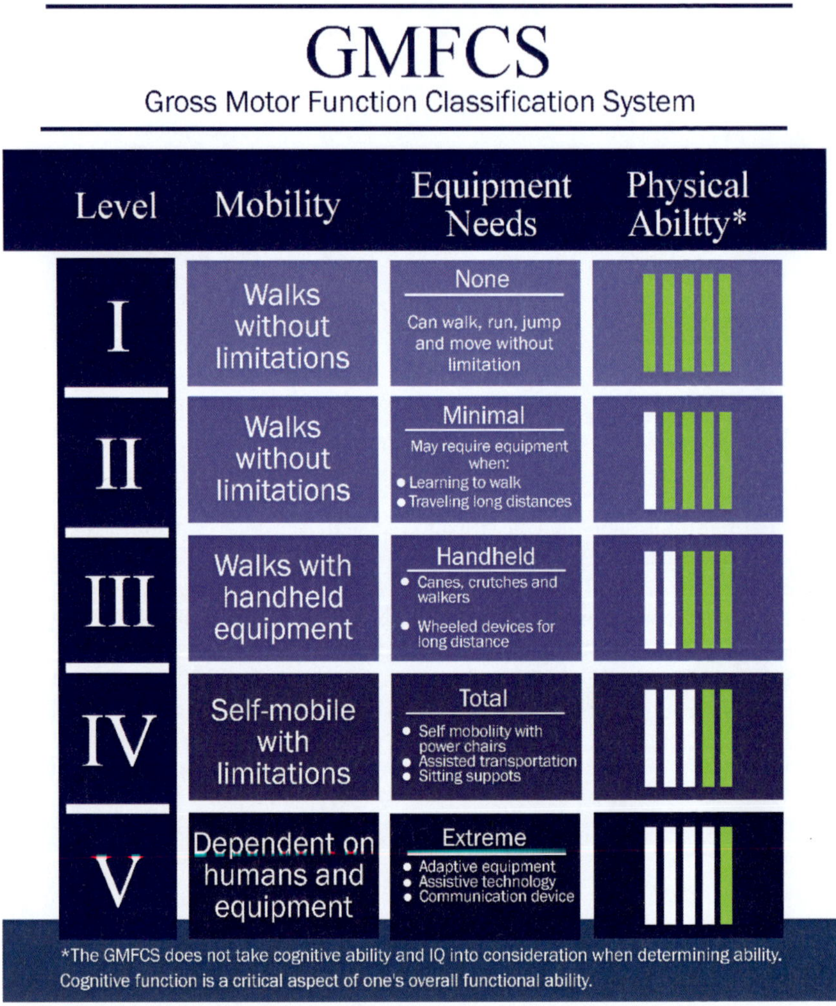

Fig. 2.11. This picture shows the Gross Motor Function Classification System (adapted from Reiter and Walsh Gross Motor Function Classification System (GMFCS), Cerebral Palsy, n.d.).

When a baby is born with such a diagnosis, it is usually unknown what the consequences are or what areas of the brain have been affected other than those visible on a magnetic resonance imaging (MRI) or computerized tomography(CT) scan. As a result, no one knows exactly what the child can and cannot do, how much he will evolve, or how far he will go. It has already been scientifically proven that the younger a person is, the greater their brain plasticity and that it declines with age (Kolb and Gibb, 2011).

A method for improving sensory and motor functions is to place children in complex environments that allow them to interact with a changing sensory and social environment and engage in far more motor activity than at home. According to research by Kolb and Gibb (2011), the most significant changes in synaptic organization can be seen when lab animals are placed in complex (so-called "enriched") environments. There have been studies that have discovered a wide range of neural changes associated with this type of "enrichment" (Greenough and Chang, 1989; Sirevaag and Greenough, 1988). A variety of sensory and motor experiences can result in long-term plastic changes in the brain. As a result, it is critical that the child's rehabilitation begins as soon as possible, and that he should be integrated into an educational institution where he can also develop his social skills.

Giving a child a variety of opportunities to experience, explore and play with the things around him is referred to as stimulation. It requires movement of the body as well as the use of all senses, particularly seeing, hearing and touching. Early stimulation is essential for a child's healthy physical and mental development. Interaction with other people and things provides natural and easy stimulation for the non-disabled child. However, it is frequently more difficult for the disabled child to experience and explore his surroundings. Extra care and special activities that provide easy and enjoyable ways to learn will be required for his mind and body to develop as early and fully as possible. The earlier a "stimulation programme" starts, the less delayed or retarded the child will be when he is older. Early stimulation programmes strive to help children become as capable, self-sufficient, happy and kind as possible (Werner, 1987, chap. 34).

CHAPTER 3

THE INTERACTION BETWEEN SPASTICITY AND PAIN

Pain and spasticity have a bidirectional relationship in the sense that they influence each other. The sensation of pain will lead to increased spasticity. Moreover, an increase in spasticity can cause a higher sensation of pain. I will give you an example to help you understand what I am talking about: assume the person diagnosed with spastic tetraparesis has pain in his hands (either in his fingers, palms, arms, forearms, biceps or his whole arm). This pain will cause muscle spasticity, which will result in increased pain.

In this book, I will use the terms pain and spasticity interchangeably, whether spasticity causes pain or pain causes spasticity.

CHAPTER 4

SYMPTOMATOLOGY

i. Facial and neck spasms

During my studies, I had a lot of pain in my face. In this way, I discovered that a lack of physiotherapy for the face leads to an increase in spasticity in this area, in the sense that the facial muscles do not relax on their own, which can lead to a growth in spasticity at the face, which, from my own experience, can be felt in the following ways:

- You feel like your whole face is burning and touching your face can be painful.
- You are having difficulty drinking, chewing and swallowing.
- You experience difficulties in articulating words correctly until the total loss of the ability to speak.
- Pain can be felt in areas close to the face (ears, eyes, nose) at a muscular level due to an increase in spasticity.
- If you frown, your forehead may hurt because the muscles in your face become spastic.

If your ability to speak is affected due to a lack of physiotherapy, you can communicate non-verbally in a variety of ways and through movements that you can make. For example, when I was in this situation, until I was able to speak again, I used my eyes to communicate with those around me: one blink of an eye meant "yes", two blinks of an eye meant "no", and my hands: lifting a finger meant "yes", lifting two fingers meant "no". Although this worked great for me, you do not have to do the same. You can try and find your own unique ways of communicating as easily as possible.

Blowing exercises, which help to strengthen the mouth, may cause uncontrolled muscle tightening or mouth twisting in children with cerebral palsy. If this is the case, DO NOT USE THEM (Werner, 1987, chap. 35).

Uncomfortable positions, like those at the dentist's office or at the hair salon, can cause neck pain and tension, which can result in increased spasticity at the neck.

A good portion of laughter, even if it is recommended, can cause increased facial spasticity and difficulty breathing during laughter. In this case, keep breathing constantly and avoid the factors that make you laugh for a while. Abdominal pain may also occur during such episodes because the abdominal muscles contract while laughing, but they remain contracted even after the person stops laughing. Also, the cold season can cause an increase in spasticity in the face, which can feel as if your face is burning or more frequently contractions in the face may occur in a shorter period of time.

ii Fighting with my hands

I used to keep my fists and hands closed as shown in Figures 4.1-4.3 until I was around 6 to 7 years old, and it required a lot of physiotherapy and patience to open my hand.

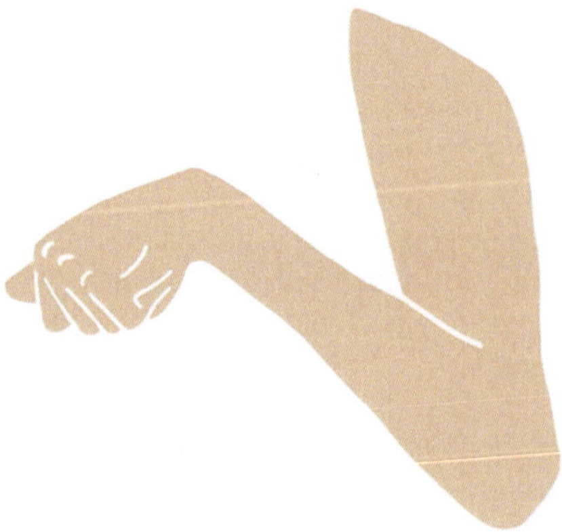

Fig. 4.1. Flexed elbow. Elbow is bent with the hand at the shoulder (adapted from NeuroGen Brain & Spine Institute, 2008).

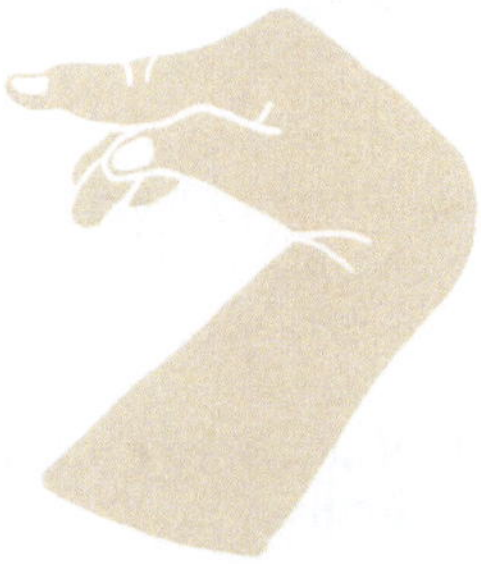

Fig. 4.2. Bent wrist. Wrist is bent with the fingers pointing down and back towards the forearm (adapted from NeuroGen Brain & Spine Institute, 2008).

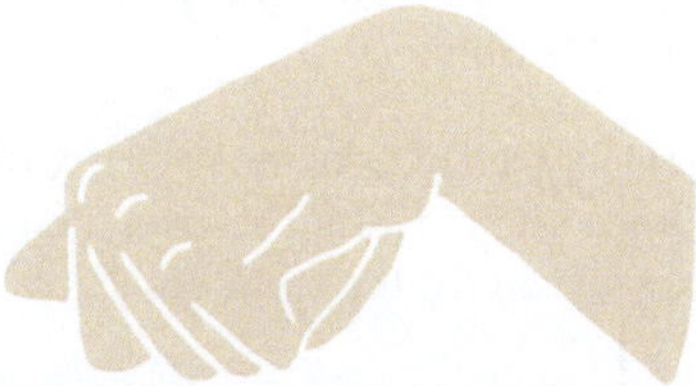

Fig. 4.3. Closed fist. The fingers are tightly clasped into the palm of the hand (adapted from NeuroGen Brain & Spine Institute, 2008).

Writing in primary school was difficult due to the fine control movement required to keep a pen in my hand. Grasping things was also difficult, as was dressing and eating by myself (holding the spoons, knives, forks and cups in my hands was painful), but with practice and therapy, my hands began to listen to me. Due to a lack of proper physiotherapy, my hands developed increased spasticity, which manifested as follows:

- Pain in the fingers, hands, wrists and palms.
- A higher difficulty in the dexterity of the hand.
- Difficulties holding a fork, cup, plate, phone, laptop, book, etc. (if spasticity worsened, difficulty turned into inability).
- Eating by myself was hard.
- Washing my hands became more difficult.
- Difficulties in taking a shower alone (see the chapter The stunning difference that the house makes for more details about how to arrange the bathroom).

- ➢ Lack of coordinated movements, which may result in items being dropped.
- ➢ Writing problems.
- ➢ Having trouble grasping things with the whole hand.
- ➢ Having trouble putting on a blouse or buttoning a shirt.
- ➢ Difficulties in the movement of supination and pronation of the hand.

Avoid keeping your hands bent under your head because doing so will increase the contractions in your arms.

Even if you occasionally experience physical discomfort when performing activities requiring the use of your hands, I recommend using both hands as much as possible in a variety of activities, as this has a positive effect on maintaining hand mobility. I often prefer handwriting over computer writing because it improves finger dexterity, allowing for a better grasp of objects, and keeps joints flexible.

According to Werner (1987, chap. 35), the majority of babies are born with a 'grasping reflex.' When you put your finger in their hand, it automatically grips it so tightly that you can lift the child up.

This reflex usually fades, and the baby gradually learns to hold and let go of objects as he pleases. Babies who are slow to develop may have little or no 'grasping reflex', making it difficult for them to learn to hold things. The following activity may be beneficial to such children. Stroke the outer edge of his hand from little finger to wrist if he keeps his hand closed. This frequently causes the baby to lift and open his hand, as well as grasp your finger (Fig. 4.4).

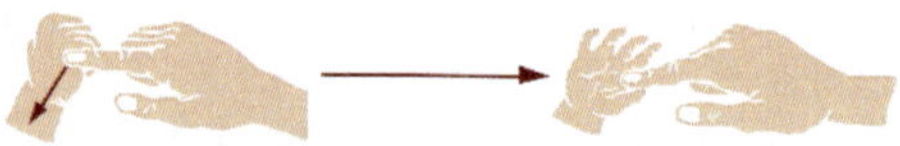

Fig.4.4. How to stroke the hand of the child (adapted from Werner, 1987, chap. 35).

When the back of the hand is stroked, a child with spasticity may grasp or open his hand stiffly and uncontrollably (Fig. 4.5). If so, avoid doing it and seek out alternatives that would give him more control (Werner, 1987, chap. 35).

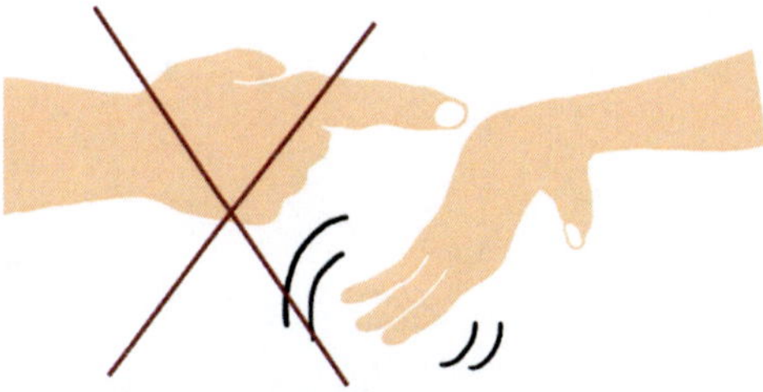

Fig. 4.5. How NOT TO stroke the back of the hand (adapted from Werner, 1987, chap. 35).

A child progresses through different stages of ability in any area of development, such as head control or hand use. For example, when a child is learning to grasp, he can first grasp with the entire hand and then with the thumb and finger (Werner, 1987, chap. 35).

Because spastic hands are more painful, muscles are always stiff, and any movement hurts.

Exercise several times per day, any type of movement, anything helps, as long as they are moved and used. The simplest one is to hold something as large as the size of your hand. You should start with this because it requires less concentration and energy. For practice, close and open your hand as many times as you want. A more difficult exercise is holding an object between the tips of your fingers. More effort and concentration are needed. As I said before, do it as many times as you want for practice. The most difficult task is to pick up and hold something small, such as a ball between two fingers, as shown in Fig. 4.6. Do it as many times as you want for practice. This is a more painful exercise but is crucial for the next steps you will take with your hands.

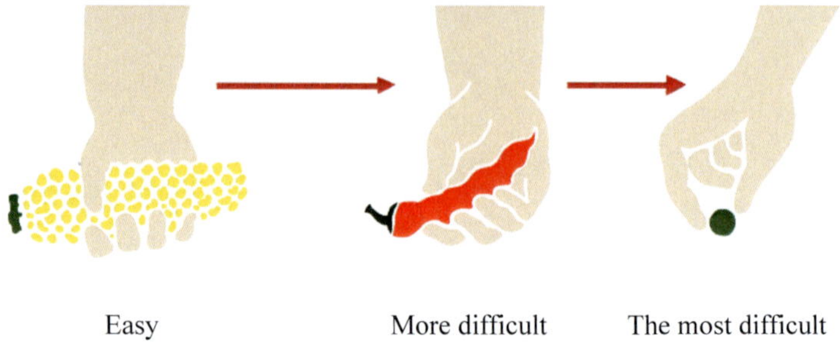

Fig. 4.6. Grasp with the entire hand and then with the thumb and finger (adapted from Werner, 1987, chap. 35).

Use your hands to guide a child's movements when helping him learn a new skill. For instance, you can teach a child to bring his hands to his mouth (or to eat by himself) by doing the following: assist him in bringing food to his mouth with a spoon in his hand as shown in Fig. 4.7. Try this activity several times until you see that the child understands the activity and then allow him to complete the task on his own. It is usually preferable to gently guide the child rather than telling him how to do something. If he tries something but has difficulty, guiding his hands so that he succeeds will make him much more eager to learn the skill than telling him "NO-do it this way!" (Werner, 1987, chap. 34).

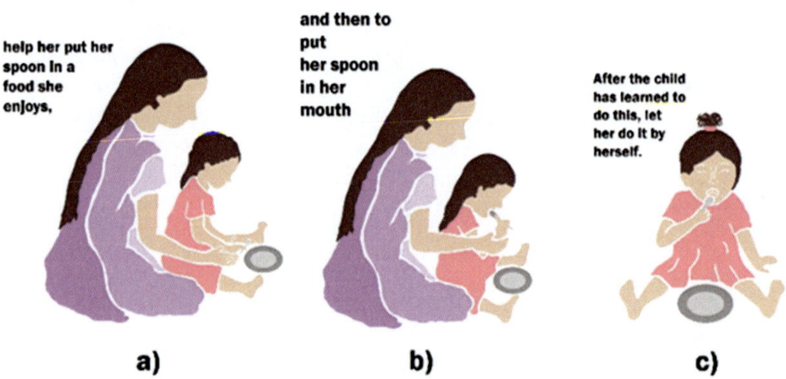

Fig. 4.7. Teaching a child to eat on his own by guiding his hands in order to bring food to his mouth (adapted from Werner, 1987, chap. 34).

iii. Leg spasticity

Children with balance issues (due to cerebral palsy, polio or another disability) frequently sit with their legs in a 'W' to avoid falling over. It is generally discouraged to sit in such a position because it can exacerbate contractures and loosen or damage hips and knees (Werner, 1987, chap. 9). When I was younger, I used to sit a lot in the W position, as shown in Fig. 4.7, and it took me a long time to correct it, but it is absolutely necessary to do so in order to be able to stretch your legs and walk later on.

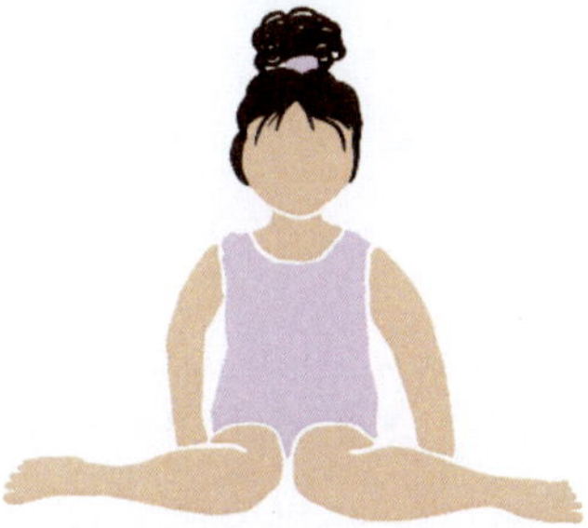

Fig. 4.7. Legs in "W" position (with the legs extremely rotated and knees flexed) (adapted from Kaur, 2017).

You can control his legs in the manner shown in Fig. 4.8. for the child with spasticity who has trouble sitting. Your hands are now free to assist him in using and controlling his arms and hands (Werner, 1987, chap. 9).

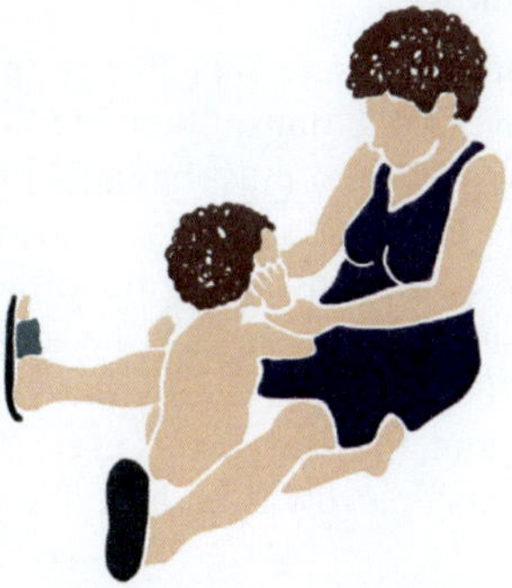

Fig. 4.8. How to position to control the legs of the child (adapted from Werner, 1987, chap. 9).

The child should be positioned on your belly with his legs extended and feet flat as shown in Fig. 4.9. As needed, provide knee support. Help him get his shoulders, arms and hands into more natural positions as he starts to reach for his face. Play a game where you hold or touch different parts of his face. FUN IT UP! (Werner, 1987, chap. 9).

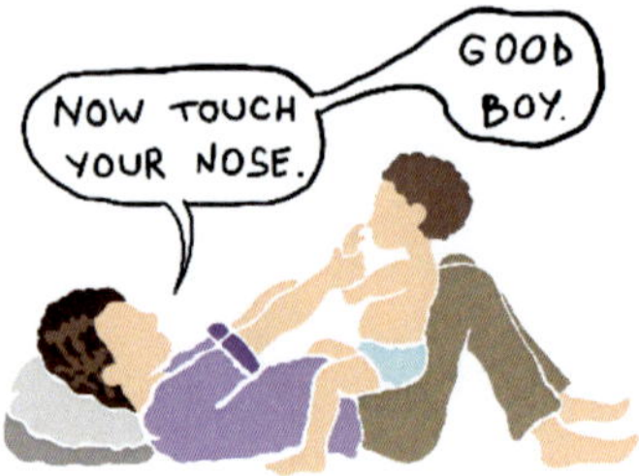

Fig. 4.9. The child is positioned on your belly with his legs extended and feet flat. As needed, provide knee support (adapted from Werner, 1987, chap. 9).

I started walking when I had the strength to stand up. Until I was 7 years old, I walked on tiptoes and was supported by my armpits from behind on both sides or by the hands in front or from the side.

I had the first operation to lengthen the Achille's tendon when I was 7, and after that, I walked on the entire sole of my foot, not just on the tips of my toes, as recommended by the orthopedist and physiotherapist. Walking was done gradually after the operation until I could put my feet on the ground and leave the weight gradually on them.

To learn how to walk and to ensure that the brain does not forget the connection and information that is transmitted from the brain to the leg in order to stimulate walking, the child must be taught to do it from an early age. It is unlikely that this information or connection can be relearned or recovered once it has been lost. Considering the orthopedic surgeon's and the physiotherapist's advice, the tendon may be lengthened or surgically intervened depending on the person's needs, but if the person loses the ability to walk or move around, the operation is useless because if the person does not walk, the tendon may narrow from lack of use.

I would like to mention that I started walking with a walking stand when I was 11-12 years old (I used a baby walker when I was younger and I also walked with support from another individual). The progress has been slow (but noticeable), and unless the person continues to move as much as possible and walk as independently as he can, the following hardships may occur:

- Difficulty in the coordination of the legs during walking or maintaining your body in balance.
- Pain (manifested either as a burning sensation, stinging or both) in the calf-leg/foot/anterior tibialis muscles or lower limb (anterior or posterior or both).
- Difficulty in stretching and bending the foot (additionally, difficulty in flexion and extension of the foot can occur). The extension becomes more and more difficult to achieve up to an incapacity to achieve this movement, which depends on the level of spasticity.
- If the person does not do physiotherapy, he may lose the ability to stand or if the spasticity increases significantly the person will no longer feel his legs.
- In the pelvis, more advanced spasticity can lead to pain during urination and/or more frequent urination than before (preferably to eliminate this option before suspecting a urinary tract infection) or to constipation. If the spasticity is worse the person may not feel when he urinates or voids.
- Peeing more frequently because the muscle is tense due to an increase in spasticity in this area and therefore the blister's capacity becomes reduced.
- Due to the hypertonia of the adductors, the knees frequently cross when walking (Gotia and Ardelean, 1993, 156) (see Chapter Surgeries).
- Hallux valgus can appear at the toes, as shown in Fig. 4.10, 4.11 and 4.12, but it also appears in other diagnoses (Gotia and Ardelean, 1993, 202).

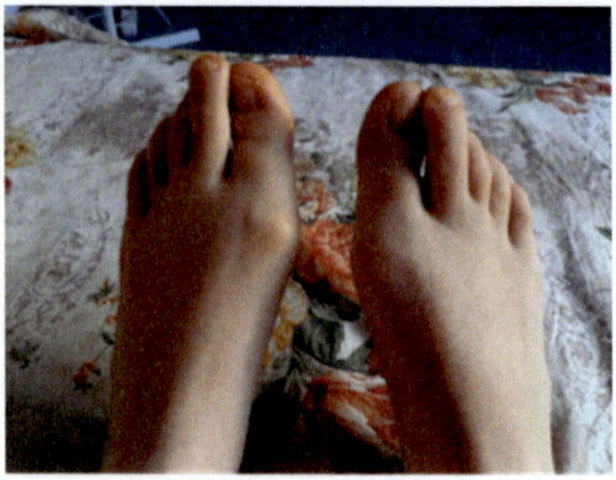

Fig. 4.10. Hallux valgus at both feet. © Bianca Wiersema. Reproduced with permission from the author.

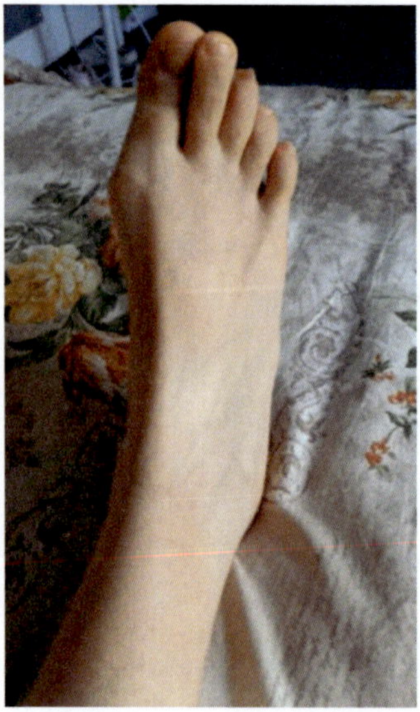

Fig. 4.11. Hallux valgus at the right foot. © Bianca Wiersema. Reproduced with permission from the author.

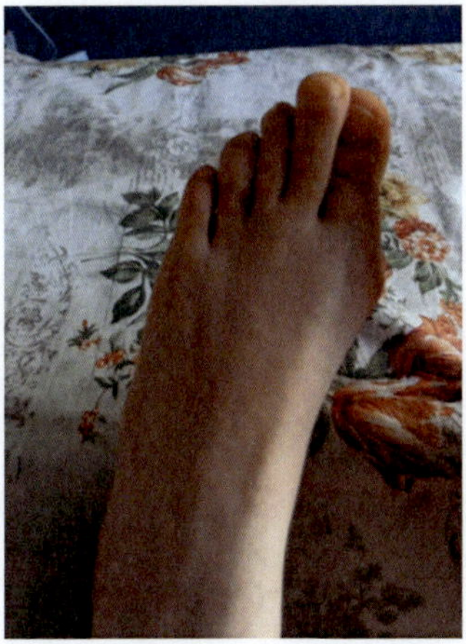

Fig. 4.12. Hallux valgus at the left foot. © Bianca Wiersema. Reproduced with permission from the author.

Leg positions

There are two major parts of a person's balance: the legs and the feet.

The legs should be parallel, and the feet should be in a normal shape.

Some of the axial deviations of the knee are genu valgum and genu varum. Genu valgum refers to the calf's deviation from the outside, while genu varum refers to the calf's deviation from the inside. Examples of genu valgnum and genu varum are shown in Figures 4.13 and 4.14 (Gotia and Ardelean, 1993, 199).

Varum's position should be solved by itself from birth to 18 months. If the child still has this problem at this age, surgery will be required.

Valgum's position - some children have it until they are one year old. If the position persists after this age, it is a sign of rickets, which usually resolves with physiotherapy. Children diagnosed with spastic tetraparesis can have genu valgum from birth, which can only be corrected with surgery as recommended by the orthopedist and ongoing physiotherapy. In this case, the person is unable to support his body weight on his feet.

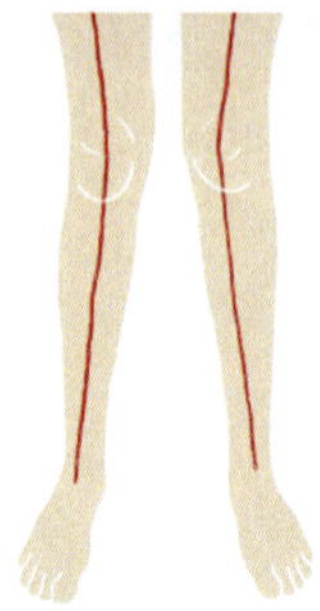

Fig. 4.13. Genu Valgnum (adapted from Bio Terra Med, "Deviațiile De Ax Ale Genunchilor (II)", Bio Terra Med, 2016).

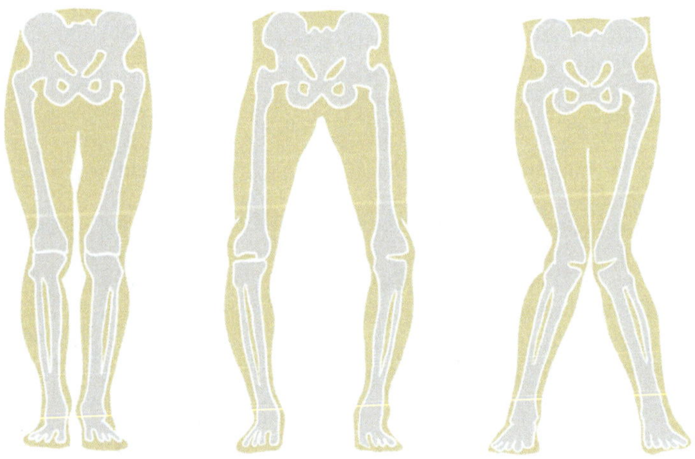

Normal position Genu Varum position Genu Valgum position

Fig. 4-14. The picture displays the Normal position, Genu Varum position, and Valgum position(adapted from Mississauga Muscle and Joint Clinic, n.d.).

Spasticity in the legs may increase during the cold season, but it may also occur during the warm season. Large temperature differences can affect the level of spasticity. Also, the person may not feel when he sweats on his feet and thus feel wet and cold (which can lead to frequent urination). As a result, wearing a pair of day and a pair of night socks can help. If a person has cold feet, the toes may stiffen and sometimes overlap one another, in addition to increased spasticity in the feet. In this scenario, the person is unable to open his toes and needs assistance to do so.

Another important point is that the person realizes with difficulty when he feels very hot or cold because the body's reactions are slower. So it is important to check how the person feels when the situation calls for it. Personally, I experience a delay in feeling when I am too cold or hot due to my slower blood circulation. For instance, I have difficulty warming up in the winter and cooling off in the summer, which may be due to my slower blood circulation.

It is not recommended to stay in the foot-over-foot position (especially when sleeping), as shown in Fig. 4.15, because one of them will rotate too far outwards (external rotation), which is not good for the correct foot position (even if it feels comfortable). Furthermore, lying like that for an extended period of time can put undue pressure on the leg that supports the other, resulting in numbness, tingling or compression.

Also, if one of the legs tends to rotate inwards too much (internal rotation), it is recommended to use a pillow placed below the knees when lying in bed in order to sit with the foot in the correct position (Fig. 4.16).

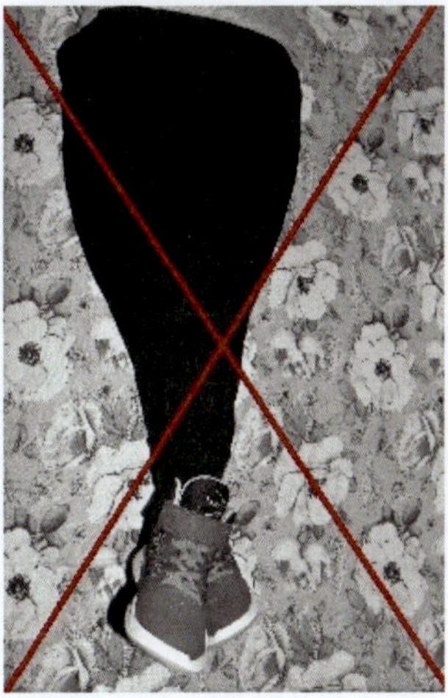

Fig. 4.15. Foot-over-foot position.

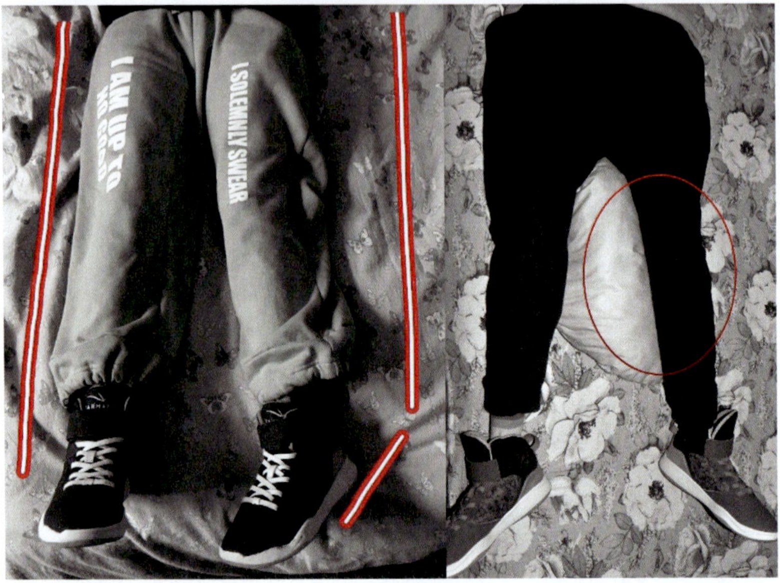

Fig. 4.16. The image on the left shows the internal rotation of the left foot and the image on the right shows the correct position of the legs, with the support of a pillow.

In the summer, I place a pillow under my heels to help my feet deflate when they swell due to the heat.

Occasionally, I use a kinesiological band to reduce internal rotation of the knee. Personally, I use the Pinotape brand, the strong therapy type band as shown in Fig. 4.17 on the left side. There are numerous alternatives that can be used (but which for me were ineffective). It is individual what kind of type you need, only together with the physiotherapist you can decide what is better for you. It is important that the tape is applied by a physiotherapist and that it is tailored to your unique needs. It is not recommended to use kinesiological tape on your own.

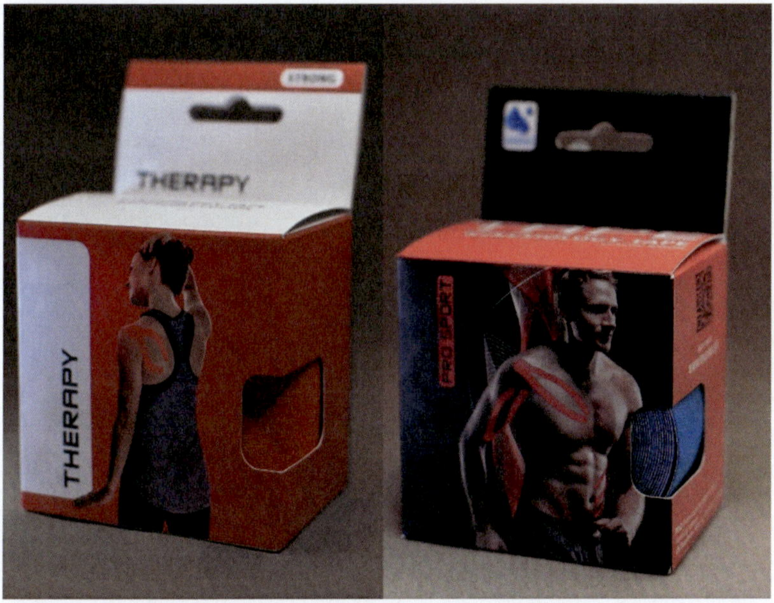

Fig. 4.17. Kinesiology tape, strong therapy type on the left side and sport type on the right side.

Some useful information about this tape:

- If it itches, burns, or stings, remove it and let your skin heal, and inform the physiotherapist who applied it to you.
- It is effective for about 2 weeks, after which it no longer has the same effect, even if it is still stuck to the skin.
- It is advised to remove it after 2-3 weeks to allow the skin to heal (the area where it was applied may be a little red-this is a natural reaction to the glue).
- If you are wearing the tape for the first time, try not to scratch in that area and give your body time to adapt.
- If improperly placed can lead to pain in the area where it is applied.
- If you buy more than two tapes at a time, the glue on them will dry out and will not stick to the body properly.
- Before applying the tape, make sure the body area where you want to glue it is clean so that it sticks better.
- It is also a good idea to leave the respective area without tape for around two weeks or more for two reasons:
  - to allow the skin to recover.

    - ❖ to learn that part to be independent and functional without the band - too much band dependence will make that area lazy.
- ➢ The tape normally lasts between 4 and 6 showers.

Parents must understand that a child develops body control and use in a specific order:

TRUNK CONTROL - HEAD CONTROL (SITTING AND BALANCE) - WALKING AND STANDING

Even an older child can confirm this. Parents of older children who are delayed, frequently try to teach them more complex skills—which children their age are learning—before they are ready. For both parents and children, this often results in disappointment and frustration (Werner, 1987, chap. 34).

I tried riding a jet ski, but it was too painful to spread my legs, and I could not open them wide enough to sit.

I tried canoeing as well, but I could not keep my balance while sitting, and my body did not react quickly enough for me to keep my balance.

iv. Abdominal spasticity

During my studies, I had a lot of stomach difficulties. After ruling out all other possibilities, The Best of the Best discovered that my issues were caused by increased abdominal spasticity, which presented in the following manner:

- ➢ Vomiting.
- ➢ Lack of appetite (or decreased appetite compared to the previous one).
- ➢ Stronger abdominal cramps while eating.
- ➢ Difficulties in emptying out until constipation.

Ingestion of fluids and food can become more difficult as spasticity increases, especially in the winter; a glass of water can easily be spilled or vomited. Abdominal pain during eating can be so severe that the person refuses to eat to avoid the pain. This leads to eating less, which leads to weight loss.

When I drink or eat, my muscles contract to digest the food, causing them to become spastic and painful, which is why I eat more slowly. If the food becomes cold as a result of taking more time to eat, the body expends more energy to compensate for the cold food and contracts. Reheating food can aid in the reduction of spasticity during feeding. Drinking tea might help to relieve physical stiffness by warming the body from within.

Consumption of plums, apples, beans or fermented foods can cause bloating, which can be painful, and thus can amplify spasticity in that area. You can try to eat them in smaller portions to avoid being bloated.

Menstrual cramps are sometimes difficult to bear during menstruation (this topic will be covered in greater detail in Chapter 5), even after taking 2-3 painkillers, which can promote spasticity. To relieve pain in the belly area, try placing something warm there, such as a hot water bottle or something else that warms the area and reduces spasticity, thereby decreasing pain.

Before taking pills to treat abdominal pain, it is preferable (and less expensive) to determine whether it is caused by an abdominal contracture which, from my personal experience, can take up to a month and a half of physiotherapy sessions to resolve, depending on how spastic the abdominal muscle is. In the case of abdominal massage, it is advised not to eat for 1 hour to 1 hour and a half after the massage to avoid vomiting. Additionally, the cold season can cause an increase in abdominal spasticity. Spicy foods should be avoided because they can amplify muscle contractions.

The sensation of evacuation is accompanied by pain rather than pressure.

If you are planning a long journey, keep in mind that you will have to stop several times because the person cannot keep himself from going to the toilet for more than two hours.

Additionally, any movement that implies getting out of a car or any other means of transport hurts. That is why some people avoid hydrating in order to avoid the pain caused by movement.

Even if the spasticity of the body decreases as a result of physical therapy, and thus the pain decreases, the person can still feel pain in the body, but it is less intense (even in a position at rest).

CHAPTER 5

SPASTICITY IN WOMEN

This section is dedicated to females, particularly to those who deal with a lot of pain during menses.

Menstrual pain can cause an increase in spasticity (at a muscular level), making the pain unbearable. I tried different drugs to ease the pain, like No-spa, but it had no effect; however, Nurofen and paracetamol were more successful. If the pain does not go away after taking the painkillers, try placing a small bottle filled with warm water in the area until the pain subsides.

Despite what you might have read on the internet about physical activity not being recommended during menstruation, I strongly encourage you to partake in it. During physical therapy certain hormones are released that can help you to relieve pain.

Those who care for someone who has her menstrual period should be aware that the person may experience the following symptoms:

- Fainting (in this case, take a wet towel with cold water and wipe the person on the face, wrists and behind the knees).

  If the person does not recover, take a towel, already sunk in with cold water and put it on the person's chest. The shock will be greater, but the person will wake up. Because of the pain, the person can scream (cold water leads to a sudden contraction of the muscles which can cause physical discomfort). If two people are standing next to the person, one can immobilize the person's hands to prevent uncontrollable hand movements during the cold water shock and to prevent others from being hit and the other can position the wet towel on various parts of the body.

- If you have one of them, give the person a tablespoon of lemon or Clorocalcin; the bitter taste can help the person wake up.

  It is important that the individual providing assistance does not panic in order to act appropriately. I suggest that you should ask the physiotherapist if applying a cold towel on the chest is advisable. A higher shock in this area leads to an increase in spasticity in this area, which can cause the person to have difficulty when breathing. Also, before the menstrual period is due, if the person feels capable, she can do one or a few more intense physiotherapy sessions (without having muscle fever). This might reduce the intense sensation of pain experienced in the first days of menstruation.

  - Diarrhea
  - Constipation
  - Bloating
  - Lack of appetite / higher appetite
  - Headaches
  - Irritability
  - Mood swings
  - Nervousness

Epilation

From personal experience, I recommend shaving with a depilatory cream rather than wax, because wax promotes muscle contractions, which can be quite painful. If you still want to use wax, try taking a Mydocalm 2 hours before to relax your muscles. (However, the effectiveness varies depending on the person).

Peeling the skin after or before shaving is not recommended in order to avoid further irritating the skin. It is also not advisable to apply tape on the leg for 3-4 days after peeling or shaving to allow the skin to calm down.

According to my personal experience, after epilation, my skin burns because of the cream, causing a sensation of pain, and this sensation can contribute to an increase in spasticity in that area. Besides, you may feel colder for the first few days after epilation, due to the lack of hair.

Permanent hair removal with a laser is an option for permanent hair removal. If you are thinking about it, talk to a dermatologist first to make sure the procedure is safe. In my case, I tolerated the procedure well and it had no effect on the level of spasticity in my body. However, in order to keep the muscles relaxed, I did physiotherapy in conjunction with this procedure. Laser hair removal in the perianal area can result in pain that spreads throughout the region and down the legs. Increased spasticity in the affected area and legs may result from this pain. Avoid using the bidet to clean after perianal epilation because the area is extremely sensitive and can cause pain. Instead, you can clean the area with a wet towel.

CHAPTER 6

THE INFLUENCE OF EMOTIONS ON SPASTICITY

When a person experiences an emotional event (either a state of happiness, anger or sadness or participates in a very exciting event such as a party or a concert), the person's body tenses, increasing its spasticity due to the emotions that he is experiencing.

As mentioned as well by Werner (1987, chap. 9) who states that when the child is upset or excited, or when his body is in certain positions, his stiffness increases. The stiffness pattern varies greatly from child to child.

Personally, and I want to emphasize this, what helps me in these situations is to inhale and exhale deeply and regularly until I manage to calm down, to allow the muscles to relax. In addition, because of muscle contractions, it is more difficult for me to breathe when I laugh too hard and for too long. Sometimes my face burns.

If there are situations in which the person has to raise his voice or scream to be heard, this will cause an increase in spasticity in the chest, resulting in difficulty in breathing. Additionally, the chest muscles will not relax after which the person returns to a normal tone, but remain tense, resulting in ongoing breathing difficulties. In this case, seek advice from your physiotherapist to resolve the issue.

The muscles tighten up when I cough, which could cause chest pain. This pain may be lessened with physiotherapy in the area.

Furthermore, it has happened to me that concentrating too hard to relax caused me to spasm even more. In this situation, focusing on anything else worked well for me. You can try to find your own way to relax yourself.

Moreover, if you intend to visit an amusement park, think about which attractions are the safest. For example, attractions without a waist belt and a base for support between the legs, such as the one shown in Fig. 6.1., are not recommended because the person may slip in front due to the spasticity that will increase, due to adrenaline.

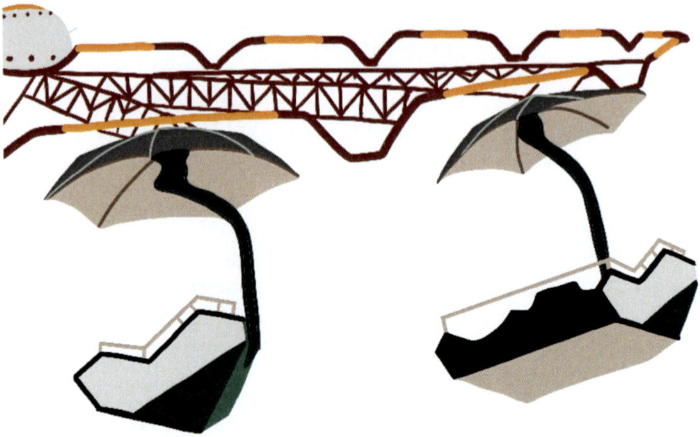

Fig. 6.1. This picture depicts an attraction lacking a waist belt and a base for support in the middle of the legs (Person, 2019).

Regardless of the challenges you face when dealing with emotional events, a portion of laughter is always welcomed.

CHAPTER 7

SLEEPING LIKE A ROBOT

Increased body spasticity can cause pain, which can affect the quality of sleep. Ideally, try not to sleep in the same position, on the same side of the body, and try to change your position at least twice a night to avoid becoming numb and in pain. I sleep in a double bed so that I can turn alone. If the bed is for one person, someone must turn the person at night, as the bed is too small to turn alone. To avoid leg pain, sleep with your knees stretched out rather than close to your chest, if you can. When lying in bed, try to hold your hands next to your body rather than under your head to avoid pain and numbness. If you keep them bent, you will favor the contractions even more. Breathing problems can have a big impact on your resting schedule. What worked best for me was physiotherapy to treat breathing problems and pain, as well as establishing a regular rest schedule. For the person diagnosed with spastic tetraparesis, the effort to carry out his activities consumes a lot more energy when compared to a person who does not have this diagnosis. As a result, the person requires more hours of sleep to rest. You can use valerian or melatonin to help you sleep, but this is only a temporary solution.

In order to prevent hurting yourself when you get out of bed, it must not have edges on the sides, as seen in Fig. 7.1.

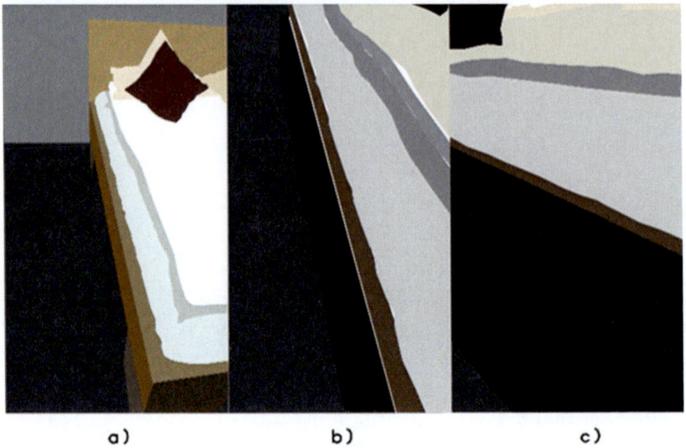

Fig. 7.1. The side of the bed has edges (which are marked in light and dark brown), which can hurt the person's leg.

CHAPTER 8

FLAT FEET AND ORTHOPEDIC HEELS

Flatfoot does not only occur in spastic tetraparesis; it can also occur in several other medical conditions (Gotia and Ardelean, 1993, 200). Wearing orthopedic heels (Fig. 8.1) may be advisable if you have flatfoot. The purpose of wearing an orthopedic heel is to create a “hole” in the feet in order to diminish the flatfoot. This may help to correct the foot position while walking.

Wearing orthopedic heels was quite painful for me (I wore about 3-4 orthopedic heels starting quite early, which were customized according to my needs at the time), especially while walking when the pain increased, which also led to an increase in spasticity in the feet. Furthermore, the heels must be adjusted according to the type of shoe you are wearing (one type of heel suits a trainer, but not a boot) and to the size of the shoe, which I will go through in greater detail in the Clothing and Footwear chapter. Furthermore, as a result of the flatfoot, the knee will tend to move inwards (Fig. 8.2.), in addition to other changes that may occur, making walking difficult. For more information about the latter, ask a physiotherapist.

Fig. 8.3. displays examples of the feet with normal, high and flat arches, which can result in a different distribution of the weight on the foot.

For me, it caused a lot of pain and it did not bring me any good results. I was walking better and straighter without these heels.

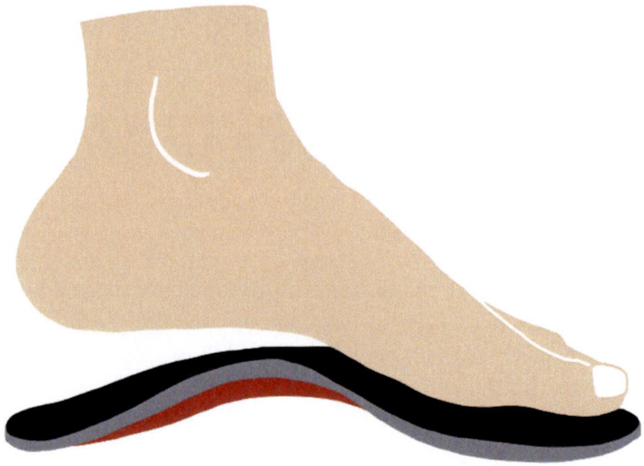

Fig. 8.1. An example of an orthopedic heel under the foot (adapted from Smartiz, n.d.).

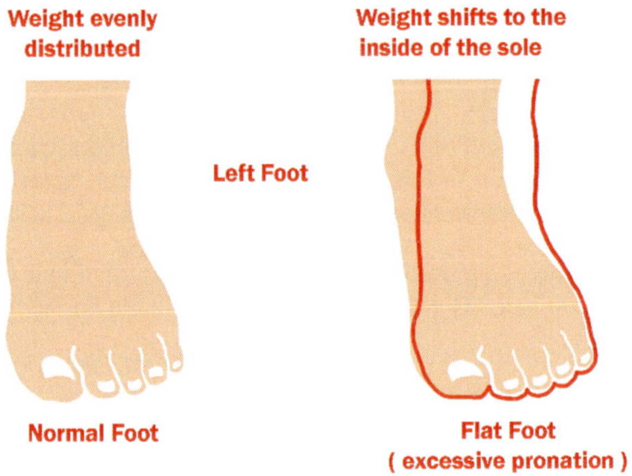

Fig. 8.2. Comparison between a normal foot and a flatfoot. A flatfoot causes a shift in the weight distribution, which leads to knees moving inwards (adapted from Flat Feet, n.d.).

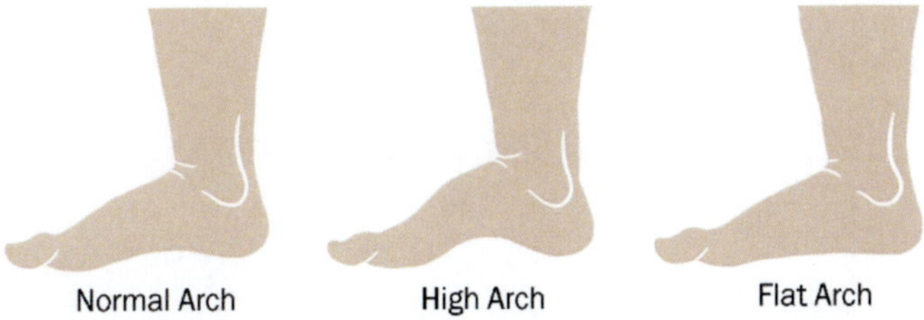

Fig. 8.3. Examples of feet with a normal, high and flat arch, which can cause a different distribution of the weight on the foot (adapted from Flat Feet vs High Foot Arch, n.d.).

You should never use the heel shown in Fig. 8.4. because the pain is excruciating.

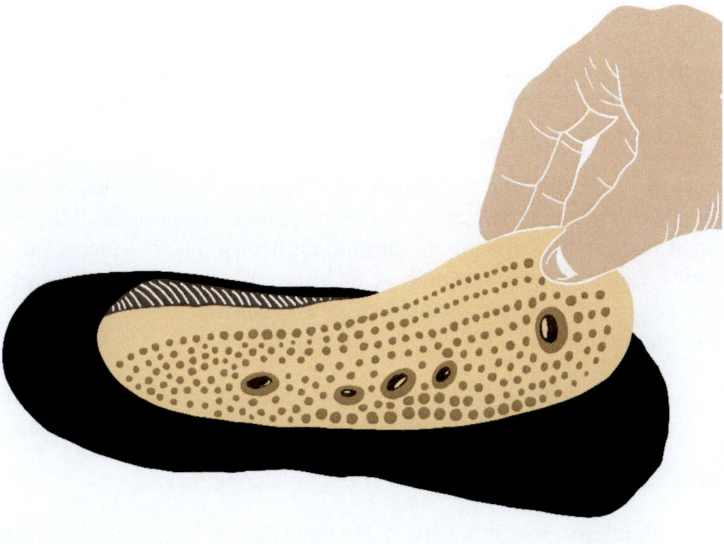

Fig. 8.4. A heel with pressopuncture (adapted from Talonete magnetice pentru presopunctura, n.d.).

CHAPTER 9

PREMATURITY AND HEARING

Premature birth can lead to an insufficient auditory system development (Nober, 1976; Stamatin, Păduraru, and Avasiloaiei, 2009). As a result, the baby may be born with a hearing impairment. If this occurs, I recommend that you consult an otologist.

Is your child experiencing difficulty hearing? Check your child's hearing if he is slow to speak. Even if he can hear some noises, he may not be able to understand speech. Furthermore, some children with good hearing may never be able to speak. Certain children with cerebral palsy, for example, are unable to control their mouth, tongue, or voice muscles. We must find other ways to communicate with these children, as we do with young deaf children (Werner, 1987, chap. 35).

Keep in mind that most children with hearing loss can learn quickly. However, some people may suffer from brain damage or disabilities that impair their ability to learn or control their hands, lips, or voices. You will need to figure out how to help these children communicate in whatever way they can: with sets of pictures, eye movements, or head movements (Werner, 1987, chap. 31).

Any child who has not heard as many words as the others, or has not heard them correctly, most likely has a hearing problem (Werner, 1987, chap. 47).

Different children have varying degrees of hearing loss

Some children are completely deaf; they cannot hear anything. Parents frequently notice that their child cannot hear early on because he does not turn his head or respond to even loud sounds. Even very loud noises have no effect on the child who is completely deaf. However, he may notice movements or vibrations as a result of sudden loud noises. Clapping behind the child's head, for example, may cause the air at his neck to move, causing the child to turn. You can try to hit the bottom of a pan with a spoon to see if he is deaf as shown in Fig. 9.1. (Werner, 1987, chap. 31).

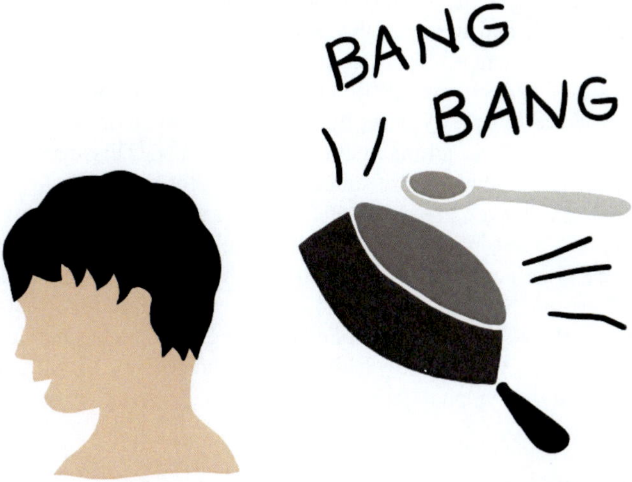

Fig. 9.1. Hitting a pan with a spoon to check if the child hears (adapted from Werner, 1987, chap. 31).

Children who are partially deaf are far more common. A child who is partially deaf hears some sounds but may not hear clearly enough to be able to distinguish between certain sounds or words. Families are frequently slow to recognize that the child is deaf. He may show surprise or turn his head in response to a loud noise, but not in response to softer noises. He may respond to low-pitched sounds such as drums, thunder, or a cow's 'moo', but not to high-pitched sounds such as a rooster crowing or a whistle. Alternatively (and less commonly), he may respond to high-pitched sounds but not to low-pitched ones. Some partially deaf children hear a little when people speak to them. They may gradually learn to recognize and respond to some words. However, they do not hear many words clearly enough to understand them. They are slow to start to speak (Werner, 1987, chap. 31). The child has some hearing if he responds to certain sounds but not others. However, he may be unable to understand language because he cannot distinguish certain words. The child frequently does not speak clearly, mixes up certain sounds, or appears to 'talk through his nose'. Unfortunately, sometimes parents, other children, and teachers are unaware that the child is deaf. They may treat him as if he is mentally slow or 'dumb'. This only enhances the child's problems. COMMUNICATION is how we understand what is said to us and how we express our thoughts, needs, and feelings to others. Speaking is the main form of communication for those who can hear (Werner, 1987, chap. 31).

Hearing and language are crucial for most growing children in learning to know, understand, and relate to the people and things around them. The most difficult challenge for a child with hearing loss is learning to communicate. It is much more difficult for him to learn to speak because he cannot hear words clearly. As a result, he has difficulty understanding what people want as well as telling them what he wants. This can result in frequent disappointments and misunderstandings for the child, as well as others. The exchange of ideas and information via some form of communication is essential for the mental development of any child, so it should come as no surprise that children with hearing loss sometimes take longer to learn how to relate to others, feel lonely or forgotten, or develop "behavior problems." The majority of deaf children are just as smart as other children. However, they need to learn to communicate well from a young age if they want their mental abilities to fully develop (Werner, 1987, chap. 31).

Early detection of deafness is crucial

A child's mind is like a sponge in the first few years of life, and they pick up language quickly. The best years for learning communication skills may be lost if a child's hearing problem is not identified early and effective help is not given (age 0 to 7). He can learn to communicate more, the earlier special training starts. Parents should keep an open eye for clues that a baby hears or not. When you suddenly make a loud noise, does the baby react with surprise or a blink? Does the infant turn his head or smile when he recognizes voices as he gets older? Has he started to speak by the age of 18 months? Is he saying a lot of words fairly clearly by the age of 3 or 4? Otherwise, he may have a hearing problem. Test the child's hearing as soon as you suspect a problem. If it appears that the child is deaf, take him to a specialist for testing as soon as possible. Deafness can be one of the most difficult, lonely, and misunderstood disabilities unless he is given a lot of understanding and help to learn to communicate from an early age (Werner, 1987, chap. 31).

For instance, a child who is deaf from birth but whose brain is normal will struggle to understand speech and learn to speak. He is consequently frequently excluded from the sharing of information and ideas. He might appear "mentally slow" for his age in some ways because language is crucial to the full development of the mind. However, if the child is taught to communicate his wishes and thoughts using 'sign language', nodding, shaking his head, or pointing (Werner, 1987, chap. 35) at the same time that other children learn to speak, his intelligence will frequently develop normally (Werner, 1987, chap. 34).

Ways to test the hearing of babies (4 months old and older)

Spending so much time with the child, parents are generally the ones who can tell if the child reacts differently to loud and soft sounds, high or low sounds. Examine whether the baby responds to his mother's voice when she is not present. The baby may react with surprise, move, turn his eyes or head toward the sound, or have no reaction at all. Alternatively, make a rattle out of seeds or small stones. Shake it behind the baby's head, first on one side, then the other (Fig. 9.2.). Check to see if the baby is surprised. Then, from various locations around the room, call out the baby's name. Take note of whether the baby responds to his name when he cannot see the person who is calling him. Check to see if the baby reacts to his name (Werner, 1987, chap. 47).

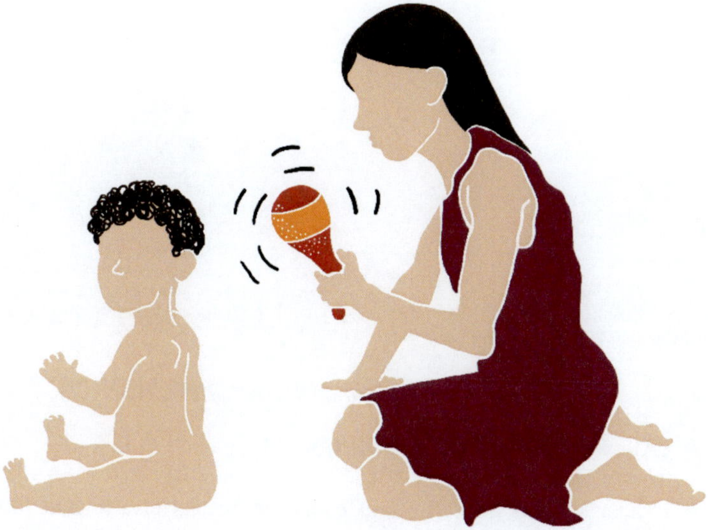

Fig. 9.2. Make a rattle out of seeds or small stones. Shake it behind the baby's head, first on one side, then the other (adapted from Werner, 1987, chap. 47).

Do this to see if a baby hears some sounds but not others. Place yourself at arm's length from the baby and to one side. Make a variety of noises when he is not looking. To test for high-pitched sounds, say "Fth" and "Ps" and then "Oooo" for low-pitched sounds. Crinkle a thin, stiff piece of paper or rub a spoon inside a cup (Fig. 9.3.) to make other high-pitched sounds. Look for other low-pitched sounds, such as a passing truck, a train whistle, a cow's 'moo,' or low notes on a musical instrument or drum. If the baby does not express surprise or turn his head in response to any of these sounds, he may have a severe hearing problem. As a result, he may not be able to speak as early or clearly as other children and will require specialized assistance (Werner, 1987, chap. 47).

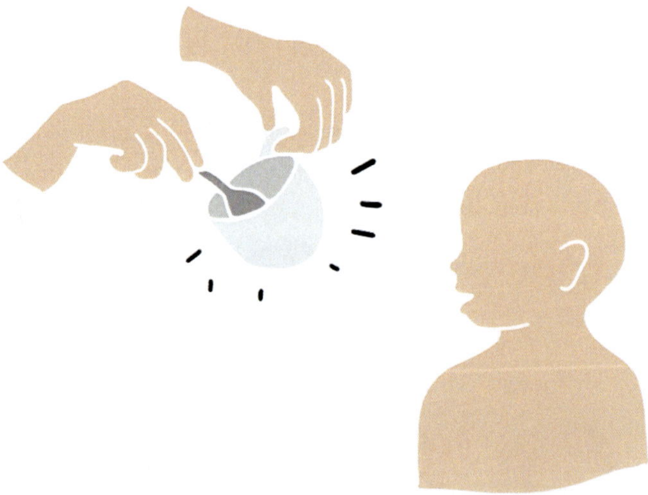

Fig. 9.3. Making other high-pitched noises by rubbing a spoon inside a cup (adapted from Werner, 1987, chap. 47).

What to do for a hearing-impaired child (Werner, 1987, chap. 47):

- Allow the child to sit near the front of the class so that he can hear better.
- Make sure in this case that everyone speaks clearly and loudly enough. But do not yell because it makes the words less clear. Check from time to time to ensure that the child understands.
- Sit one child who hears well next to the child who hears poorly, so that things can be repeated and explained as needed.
- Always make an effort to look at the child while speaking to him.
- If possible, the child should be examined by a health professional, especially if he has pus in his ears, or suffers from frequent earache.

Improving a child's hearing

Sometimes it is possible to help children who are not completely deaf to hear better. When possible, have a specialist examine the child's hearing and ears. A few children are born with a closed ear tube or another ear structure defect. These issues are rarely corrected surgically, and the children can hear better as a result. (Note: surgery will not help children whose hearing loss is caused by brain damage).

Children who have hearing loss due to ear infections may begin to hear better if they are treated early and preventative measures are taken. Some children benefit from hearing aids that make sounds louder. A hearing aid helps some children understand words and can make a significant difference in learning to listen and speak. For other children, an aid increases their awareness of sounds (which is beneficial), but it does not help them distinguish between words. If it appears that the child will benefit greatly from a hearing aid, it is best to start as early as age one or two (Werner, 1987, chap. 31).

There are various types of hearing aids available, depending on the child's level of hearing. A battery-powered hearing aid is preferable (for some children), but not for others. These, however, are usually very expensive. It should be fitted by a specially trained worker after the child's hearing has been thoroughly tested. Ask for instructions on how to keep the hearing aid clean, dry, and functioning properly if you buy one for him. Make sure you have a supply of extra batteries at hand and are aware of where to find more (Werner, 1987, chap. 31).

Young children who have difficulty hearing can sometimes be helped to listen more carefully and learn to distinguish between sounds. Make various noises and encourage the child to pay attention. "Listen to the donkey," or "What was it?" say clearly and loudly when a donkey brays or a baby cries. Praise the child if he responds or points in the right direction. Try also hitting pans, drumming, ringing bells, and so on. Examine his ability to move or dance to the beat of music or drums. Talk to the child a lot. Also, sing to him. Tell him the names of various parts of his body and other details. Request that he touches or points to them. When he does, compliment him. To get a child's attention or get him to imitate your sounds, experiment to determine how close you need to be and how loud you need to speak. Attempt to speak loudly and close-by after that. Speak loudly but without shouting.

It is best to wear hearing aids as soon as you become aware of the problem. If you find out too late, there is a chance the child will not recover completely from the hearing loss because the auditory nerves are not being stimulated to develop.

In my case, my parents discovered I could not hear when I was 7-8 years old when they noticed I was not responding to what they were saying to me, especially when they were talking behind me. The sooner you discover it, the sooner you can take action and avoid screaming or the feeling that the child does not listen because he cannot hear you, and not because he does not want to. I had to do speech therapy as a result of the fact that my parents found out so late that I could not hear.

If he wears hearing aids that suit his needs, allow time for him to adjust to the sounds he hears and provide an explanation for them, such as the noise when water flows from the tap, so that he can discover the meaning of various sounds. For someone who has never heard, the high level of sounds can make him feel disoriented, confused, and, at first, scared by everything he hears. It is a completely normal reaction, and the key to dealing with this change as smoothly as possible is to remain calm and patient and explain each sound because they are new and he has not heard them until now.

During the pandemic, I had to wear a mask to protect myself. However, this prevented me from reading people's lips. Even though I wore hearing aids, I unconsciously kept looking at people's lips as confirmation that what I was hearing was correct. What can I say, old habits die hard. This made it difficult for me to hear what others were saying, and there were moments when I believed I could not hear anything except background noises. Because of that I ended up frowning as a reaction to trying to understand what others were saying. To help overcome this difficulty, the person's family can wear a mask while speaking to the person, allowing him to hear rather than focus only on lip reading. Sometimes, I feel dizzy and nauseous if I do not wear my hearing aids for a while.

CHAPTER 10

STRABISMUS

Premature birth can result in vision problems like myopia, premature retinopathy, and strabismus as shown in Fig. 10.1. (Stamatin, Păduraru, and Avasiloaiei, 2009). It is not clear whether strabismus is unique to spastic tetraparesis. If not treated in time, surgery is necessary, which, when combined with a diagnosis of spastic tetraparesis, can make recovery extremely difficult (especially when the muscles of the face and eyes contract, the pain will be even greater, in addition to the pain of the surgery itself). Please consult a doctor, who will advise you on the best course of treatment.

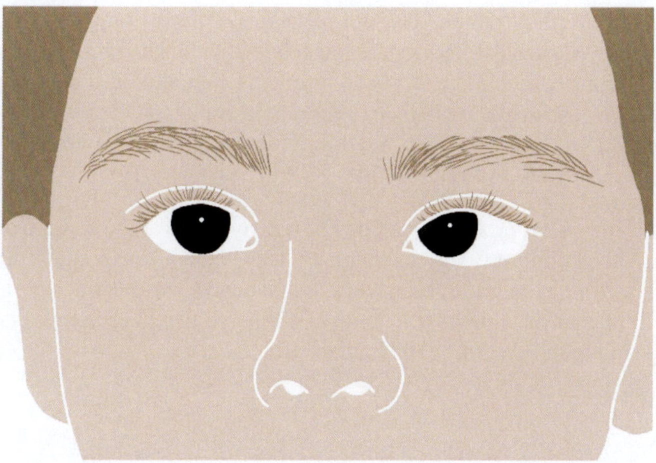

Fig. 10.1. This image depicts a child with esotropia, a type of strabismus. The left eye of the child turns inward toward the right eye (adapted from Strabismus, n.d.).

Before the surgery, try the following exercises (the sooner you start the better your chances will become of not needing the surgery):

- ➢ Take pencils, crayons, or something else that will catch the child's interest and have him follow the item as you move it from left to right or vice versa.
- ➢ If the child is capable, make him read something he would enjoy (in this way you will teach him to focus and train his eye muscles).

Strabismus (as well as flat feet) can even occur in full-term babies.

I corrected mine with a lot of exercises since I was very small, my mum used colourful toys, pencils, anything that I liked and I had to look after them. I discovered that I had vision problems at school when I could not read the letters on the blackboard. Also, I could not read the small print in books, and I got tired or headaches a lot while reading.

One of the consequences of spastic tetraparesis is partial blindness or less partial vision, which can be caused by, among other things, the child being exposed to oxygen in the incubator with unprotected eyes—it is well known that oxygen attacks sight (Tin and Gupta, 2007; Hartnett and Lane, 2013). —and thus going blind, or by prematurity, which caused a partial loss of sight. Cerebral palsy patients are not necessarily blind; some simply have poor vision. If partial blindness is detected after birth, or if it was not detected because the blindness/vision problems were minor, parents can be cautious when playing with their children, stimulating their vision with colours and movements, and watching to see if their children follow commands (Werner, 1987, chap. 30).

A child with vision problems can develop early skills at the same rate and level as other children. He can learn to feed, bathe, dress, and care for himself, as well as to walk home without assistance. Despite his inability to see well, he can develop an exceptional ability to use his senses of smell, hearing, and touch (Werner, 1987, chap. 30).

CHAPTER 11

TOOLS TO INCREASE YOUR INDEPENDENCE

A. My buddy, the wheelchair

The wheelchair might be your best friend or your worst enemy. Choosing the wrong one can make your life a nightmare. To determine what features the wheelchair requires, think about its purpose and the needs of the person who will be using it.

When I was younger, I used to wear a belt or scarf around my waist, while sitting in a chair, to prevent me from sliding forward as shown in Fig.11.1. The knot was tied on the back of the chair so that it did not hurt my abdomen. When I could sit up straight on my own, my parents stopped using the belt.

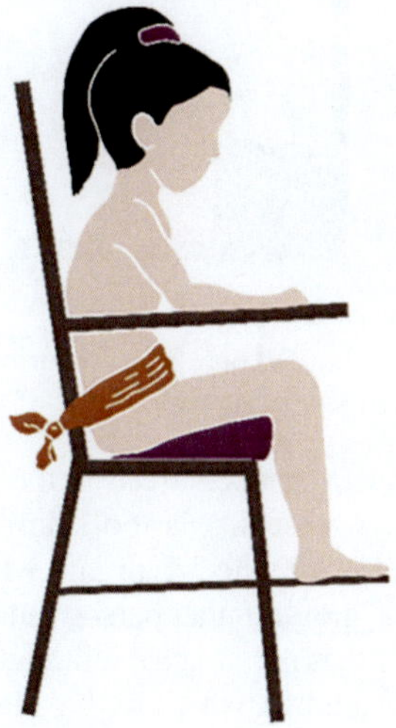

Fig. 11.1. This picture shows how to wear the belt around the waist correctly (adapted from Werner, 1987, chap. 64).

A high hip strap will not help if the person's hips are tilted back like in Fig. 11.2. In this situation, a low hip strap helps in maintaining an appropriate hip angle (Werner, 1987, chap. 65).

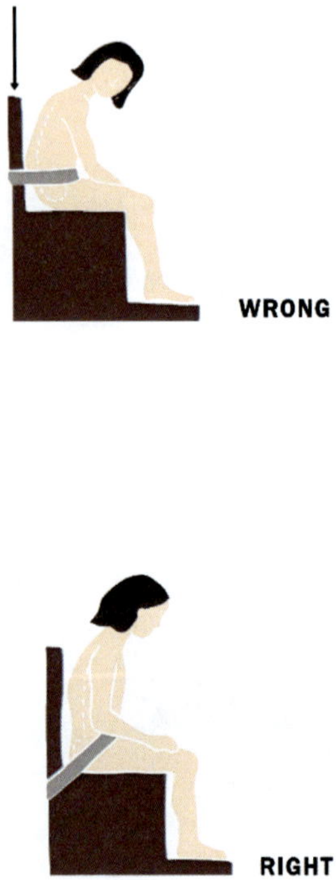

Fig. 11.2. This picture shows how to put the strip correctly if the person's hips tilt back (adapted from Werner, 1987, chap. 65).

When choosing a wheelchair, make sure it is the right size for the person who will be sitting in it. A seat that is too small will make it difficult to properly place the person in the wheelchair and will restrict the movements of the individual that is moving the person and the one sitting in the wheelchair. A wheelchair that is too large will cause the person who sits in it to lose his balance and stability, which will lead to pain in the back and in the legs. This can affect the level of spasticity of the body.

I used the template shown in Fig. 11.3. to determine the best size of the wheelchair for me, which was provided by Southwest Medical company, which recommended Joshua Dickerson to me.

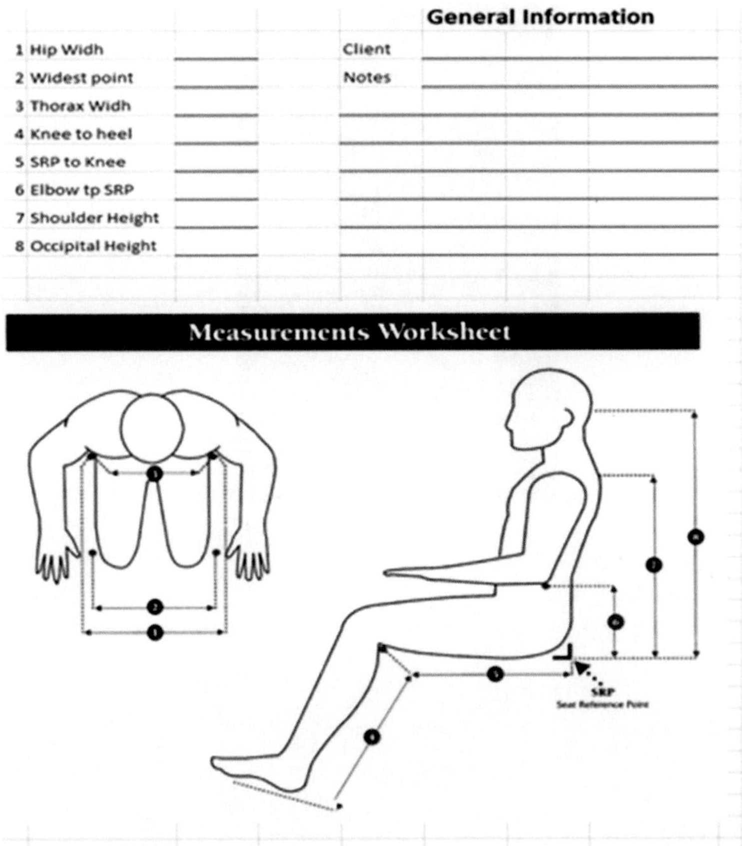

Fig. 11.3. Measurement Worksheet to help decide the right size for the wheelchair. Reproduced with permission from Joshua Dickerson.

It is critical that the wheelchair has a good braking system (Fig. 11.4.) and a pillow designed specially for long periods of sitting in the chair to avoid pain in the buttocks (I prefer the Jay Cushion because it already has a shape for the legs and buttocks, making it easier for me to position myself correctly; see Fig. 11.5.). To avoid sliding off the wheelchair make sure that the feet are supported by the footrest, which provides stability and comfort, also preventing leg pain. I often use a band in front of my legs to keep them from sliding and to provide stability. I suggest using a footrest with a band behind the heels to prevent hitting your heels at the wheels, as shown in Figures 11.6. to 11.7.

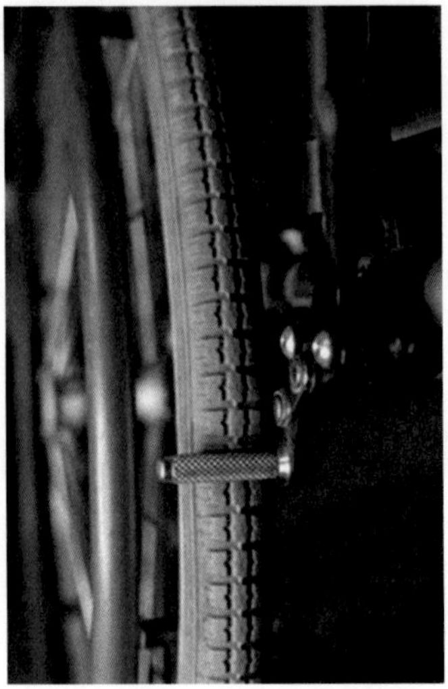

Fig. 11.4. Braking system.

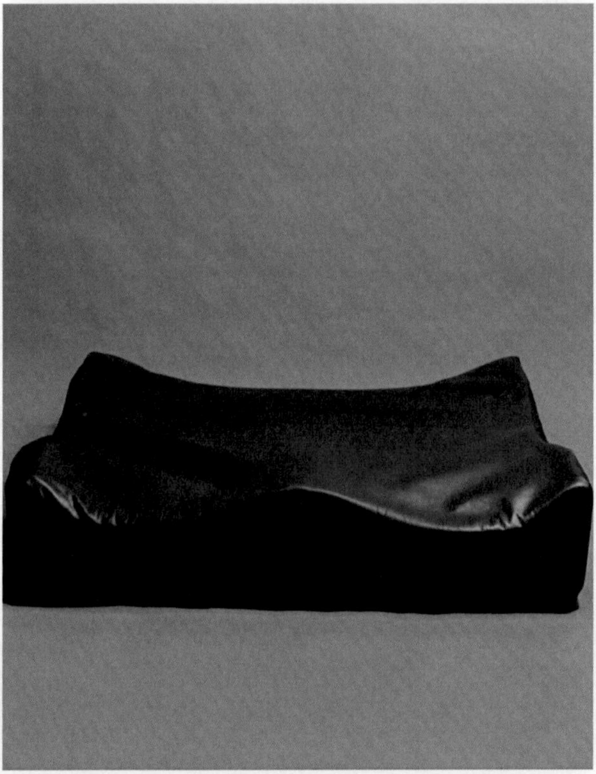

Fig. 11.5. Jay Cushion pillow that has a shape for the legs and buttocks.

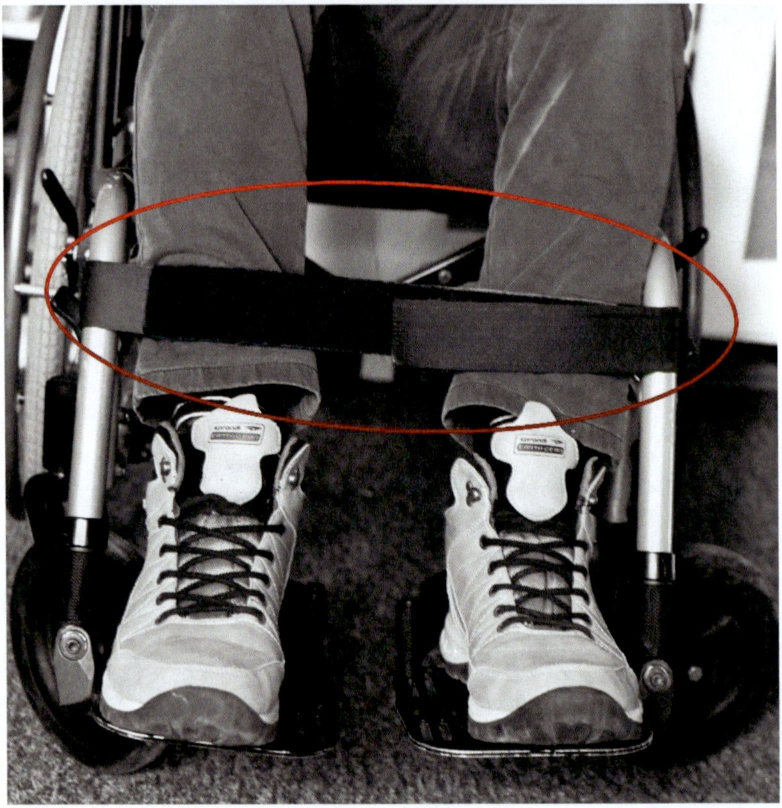

Fig. 11.6. Band to prevent the legs from sliding to the front.

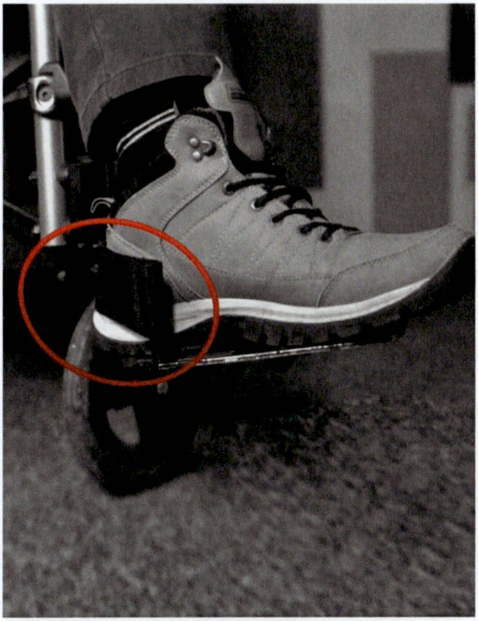

Fig. 11.7. Footrest with a band behind the heels.

Footrests that are too far forward, causing the knees not to bend enough, can also increase spasticity, tilting the hips back (Werner, 1987, chap. 64). A person can slide forward if he is seated with his legs bent beyond 90 degrees. He runs the risk of leaning forward and falling if he sits with his legs bent less than 90 degrees.

A good position is frequently achieved through the following elements: a fairly stiff, upright back at a right angle to the seat, a chair that fits the child so that his hips reach the chair back, knees at right angles (at about 90 degrees), and feet firmly supported (see Fig.11.8). Most children, particularly those who tend to fall forward in their seats, will sit better and more comfortably if the entire chair is slightly tilted back (see Fig. 11.9.). However, keep right angles at the hips, knees, and ankles (Werner, 1987, chap. 64).

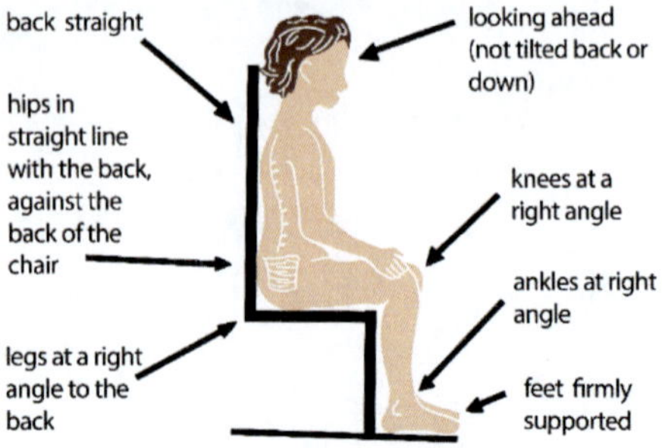

Fig.11.8. A good position in the chair (adapted from Werner, 1987, chap. 64).

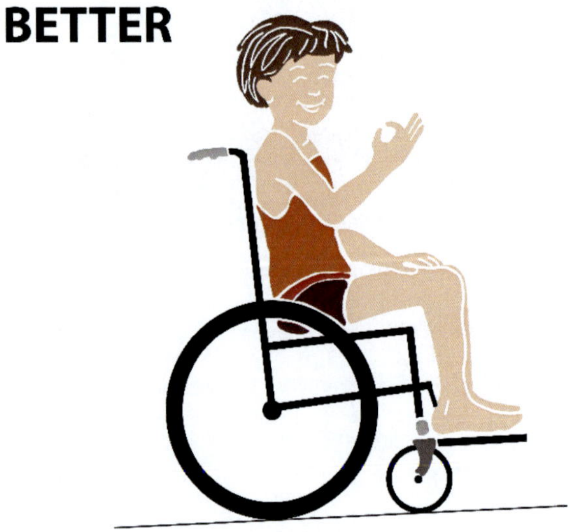

Fig. 11.9. A good position in the wheelchair (adapted from Werner, 1987, chap. 64).

I added the following items to my wheelchair to make sitting more pleasant and comfortable:

- Armrest (see Fig. 11.10.).

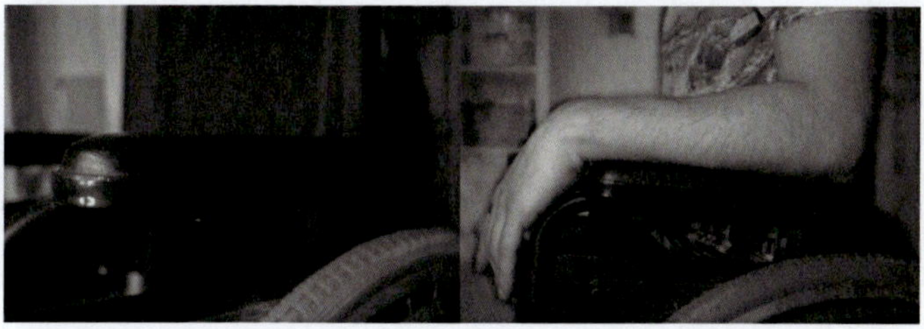

Fig. 11.10. Armrest position.

- When you are in a public place and need to write, a comfortable table (see Fig. 11.11.) is essential (conferences, work, etc.)

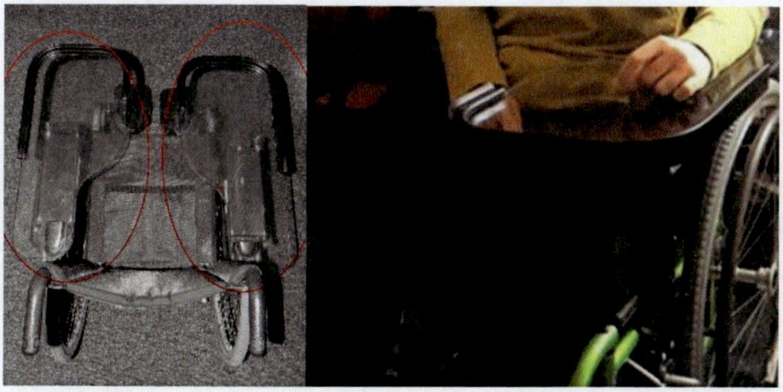

Fig. 11.11. Arm tray connected to the armrest.

- When it comes to the wheels, the back ones have pneumatic tires, while the front wheels are full but I recommend having them pneumatic too; wheels with air have a higher shock absorption than other types of wheels (Fig. 11.12. and 11.13.).

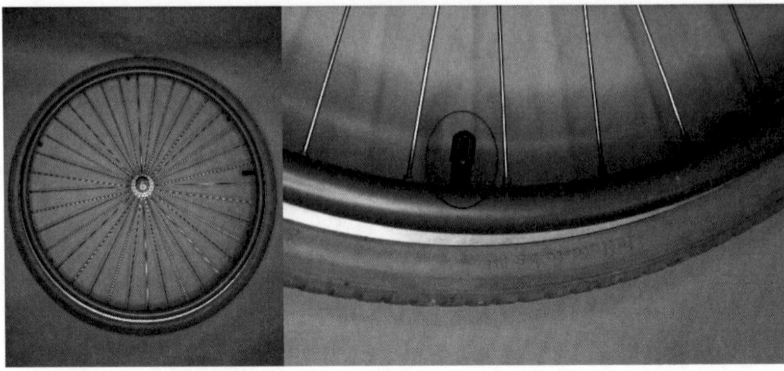

Fig. 11.12. Pneumatic back wheel.

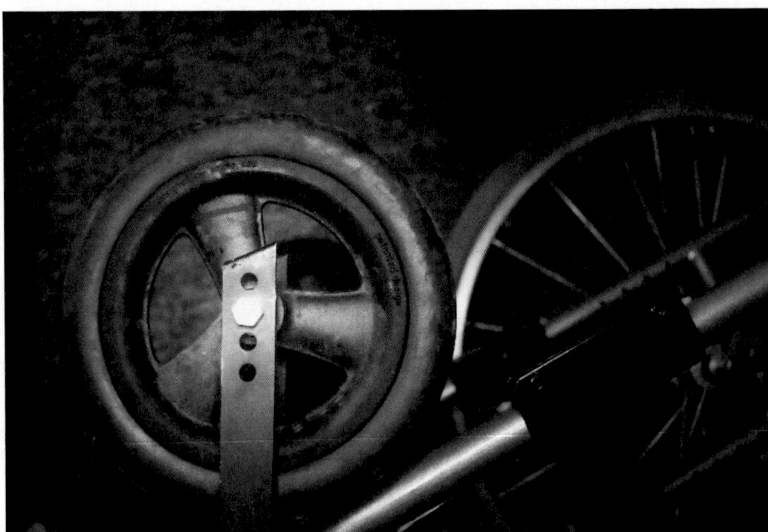

Fig. 11.13. Full front wheel.

If you can use your upper body, a wheelchair without an armrest may be a better option for you (Fig. 11.14).

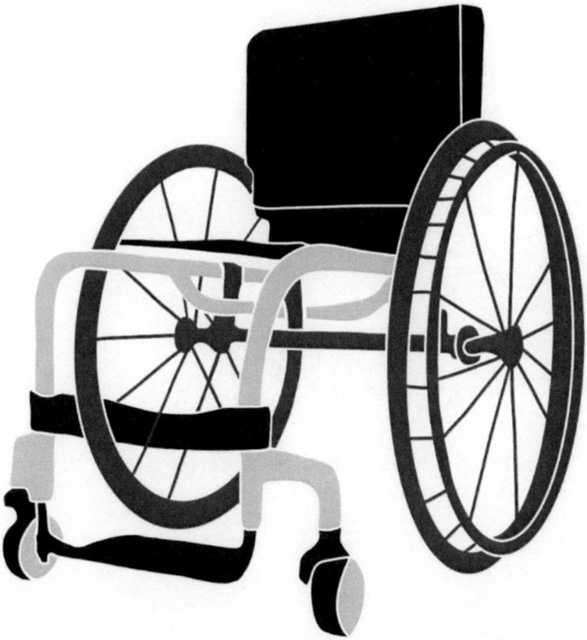

Fig. 11.14. This picture depicts a wheelchair without an armrest (adapted from SunriseMedical, n.d).

Electrical wheelchairs with joysticks are also available, which may be suitable if you have sufficient mobility in the arms and reduced spasticity in your hands, but in the worst-case scenario, the wheelchair's battery will die when you need it the most.

I am not able to use a wheelchair with a joystick because the position of my hand needed to control the joystick (Fig.11.15), could lead to spasticity. A joystick requires dexterity of the hand to coordinate precise movements and react on time. In my situation, there is a delay in the reaction due to the fact that information regarding the action that needs to be executed takes more time to be processed.

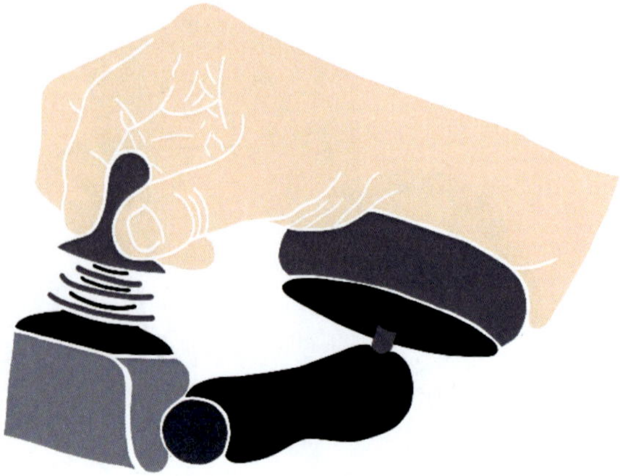

Fig. 11.15. This picture illustrates a joystick and the position of the hand (adapted from Linds Rehabilitation Equipment, n.d.).

If you plan to use your wheelchair mainly outside, choose one with a bigger wheel diameter of the front and back wheels; this will make the ride more comfortable and easier for you.

I would like to point out that for someone diagnosed with spastic tetraparesis, pushing the wheels with their hands can have a negative effect on their hands. It can lead to increased spasticity in the biceps, arm, forearm, and triceps, which will lead to poorer hand coordination and quite intense pain in the hands.

From my own experience, after a week in a camp with people who had a different diagnosis of diplegia and paraplegia than mine, a week in which they made me push the wheels of the wheelchair in order to increase my independence, even though I could not and they were aware of my limitations, it took me nearly a month and a half of physiotherapy to recover what I had lost in that week. By forcing people with different diagnoses to do the same thing despite their differences, you risk making them feel worse and humiliated. If you want a person with a certain diagnosis to do something, make sure that he is placed in a group of people with the same diagnosis, so that they feel equal.

Paraplegics can push with their hands on the wheels because their upper limbs are not affected. I want to emphasize that a person diagnosed with diplegia or paraplegia will have different abilities and limitations than a person diagnosed with tetraparesis, and the wheelchair must be adapted to each person's mobility and limitations. Do not push a person's boundaries, as you may end up doing more harm than good (a person with spastic tetraparesis will not be able to push the wheels of the chair no matter how much the people around him would like that, compared to someone diagnosed with diplegia or paraplegia).

A cheap wheelchair is generally unsuitable for this diagnosis because it lacks comfort and cannot be adjusted sufficiently to meet the person's needs. In general, these wheelchairs are heavier and more difficult to push, making life much harder for the individual pushing or lifting the wheelchair. The wheelchair is one of the things that you should not buy cheaply because a person's life revolves around it.

I contacted Joshua Dickerson about my wheelchair; more information about what they offer can be found on their website[2]. Joshua designed the wheelchair based on my needs and took into account all the information to provide me with the best wheelchair that met my needs. I can honestly say that he did his absolute best, and I am very pleased with his services; if you need someone who is dedicated to his job, and pays close attention to detail, I recommend him.

When I was younger, I was transported in structured carriers, which caused me physical discomfort because I could not spread my legs wide enough and had to sit in one position for an extended period of time, facing the person who was carrying me. Using structured carriers to transport a baby more easily is quite painful for the baby if he sits with his face toward the person who is carrying him because his legs must be spread open (if the baby is sitting with the legs together and not open) and pain in the bottom and back may occur as a result of the baby sitting in one position for an extended period of time. Instead, try to place the baby forward to encourage him to open his legs less, and massage his bottom and back on a regular basis to relieve pain.

Avoid carrying the child in the manner shown in Fig. 11.16. if he typically lies with his legs straight and arms bent. Carry him so that his arms are straight and his knees and hips are bent, as depicted in Fig.11.17. You can support him less as you carry him as he develops more self-control (Werner, 1987, chap. 9).

---

[2] https://www.southwestmedical.com/.

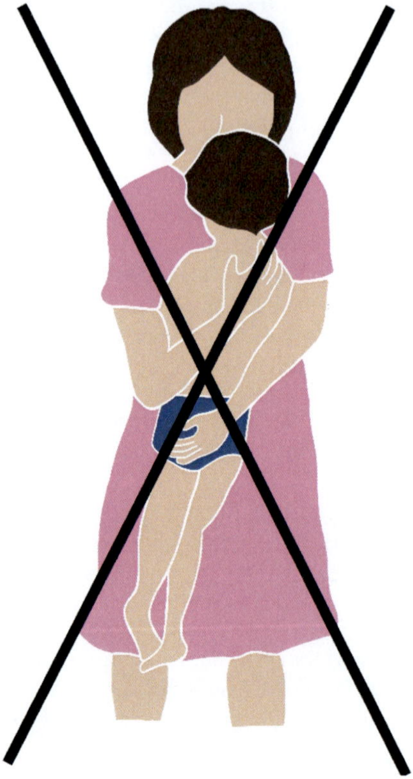

Fig. 11.16. If the child usually lays with his legs straight and his arms bent, avoid carrying him in this manner (adapted from Werner, 1987, chap. 9).

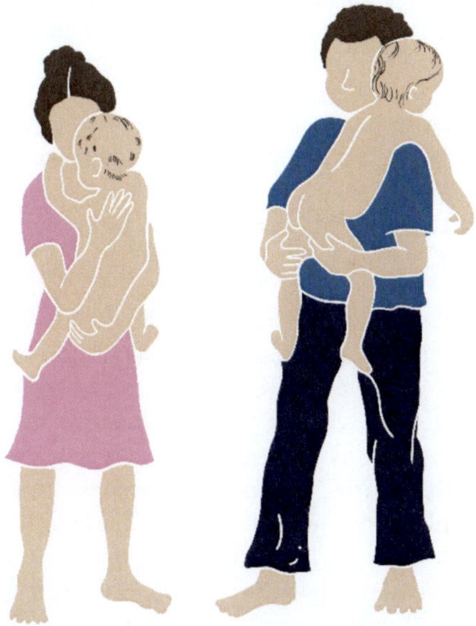

Fig. 11.17. This image shows how to carry the child with his arms straight and his knees and hips bent (adapted from Werner, 1987, chap. 9).

Backless chairs are not recommended because the person can lose his balance and move around, increasing the risk of falling from the chair. Using chairs with wheels is frequently difficult because the chair is unstable while on wheels and can move while the person is attempting to sit in it, potentially resulting in the person falling while trying to sit down. A chair with a backrest and arms is the most secure. It is preferred for the chair to be flat and soft with cushion material because it aids in finding balance when sitting on the chair. Straight-back chairs are the most recommended because they help support the back's straightness.

B. Wheelchair and car transfer

In this chapter, I will go over the transfer methods I use when I need to be moved from one location to another. Out of all my attempts, the transfer methods that worked the best for me are described below (there are several transfer methods and you can search for them and see which one suits you best).

To avoid overloading the upper body muscles of the individual performing the transfer, the weight is shifted to the lumbar area and to the legs. To avoid discomfort, both individuals must lift the person at the same time.

This approach seemed to be the least demanding for both me and those who made the transfer if there are two people who can make the transfer (but it is not universally valid). The person being transferred must sit on his bottom, preferably with his legs bent, but this technique can be used with his legs outstretched as well.

In order to transfer someone, the individual should position himself behind the person and place his arms under the shoulder while grabbing the forearms of the person being transferred as depicted in Fig. 11.18. Ask the person you are transferring whether you are squeezing the forearm too hard or if it is comfortable. To avoid your hands slipping during the transfer, make sure you have a firm grip on the person's forearms. The other individual should place his arm under the knees of the person being transferred, while the person will rest both legs on his hand. Ask the person if he feels comfortable in this position. Both individuals should pick up the person who is being transferred at the same time and move to the place where the person has to be, in a coordinated manner. Some people may be concerned about being transferred for a variety of reasons. If this is the case, speak with the person who is being transferred about the movements that you are going to make.

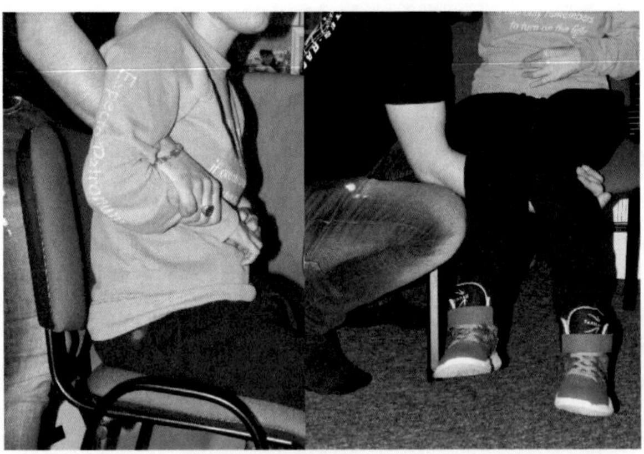

Fig. 11.18. The picture on the left shows how to grab the arms and on the right how to grab the legs when transferring the person.

If only one individual is transferring the person, the individual should position himself behind the person and place his arms under the person's shoulder while grabbing the forearms of the person being transferred (Fig. 11.18). Then, lift the person and move him to the desired location.

Personally, when I need to make a transfer in the car, I use one of the two methods described below, depending on how easy it is for me. The door is opened as wide as possible and the distance between the car and the ground should be as low as possible. Avoid vehicles with high ground clearance. Fig. 11.19., Fig. 11.20., and Fig. 11.21. demonstrate how to get into the car.

In the first method, I begin by sitting on the edge of the car seat with my feet on the ground for stability, and I grab something stable with my hand to ensure my balance. When I am stable, the individual grabs my left leg and bends it before placing it in the car. Following the placement of the first leg in the car, the individual performs the same maneuver with the other leg. After both my feet are in the car, the individual pushes my pelvis into the car so that I can sit comfortably as illustrated in Fig. 11.20.

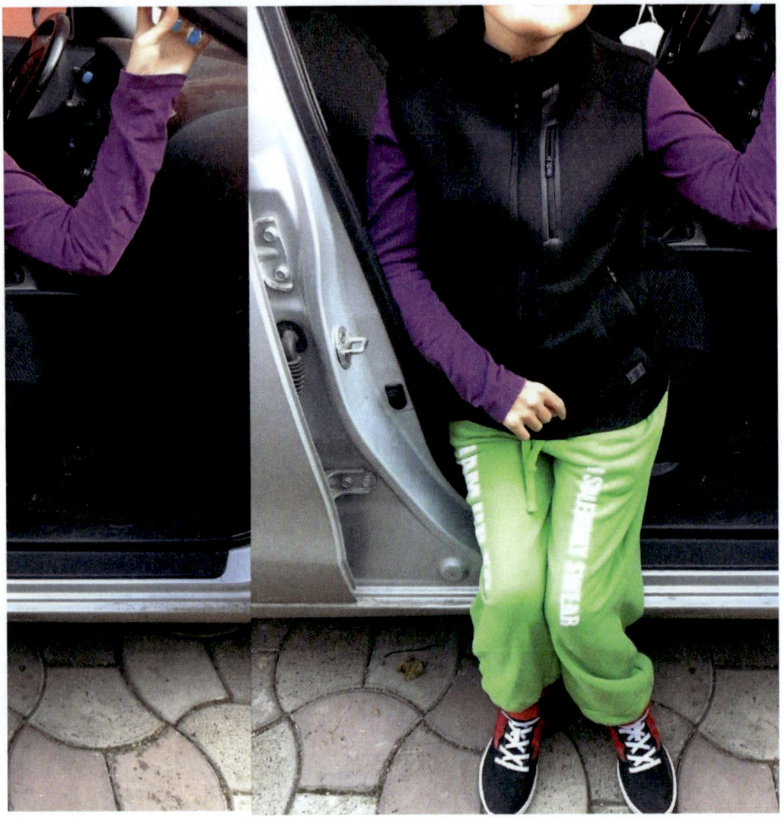

Fig. 11.19. The picture on the right shows how to position your feet on the ground, and the picture on the left how to grab something in order to make sure you are stable. © Bianca Wiersema. Reproduced with permission from the author.

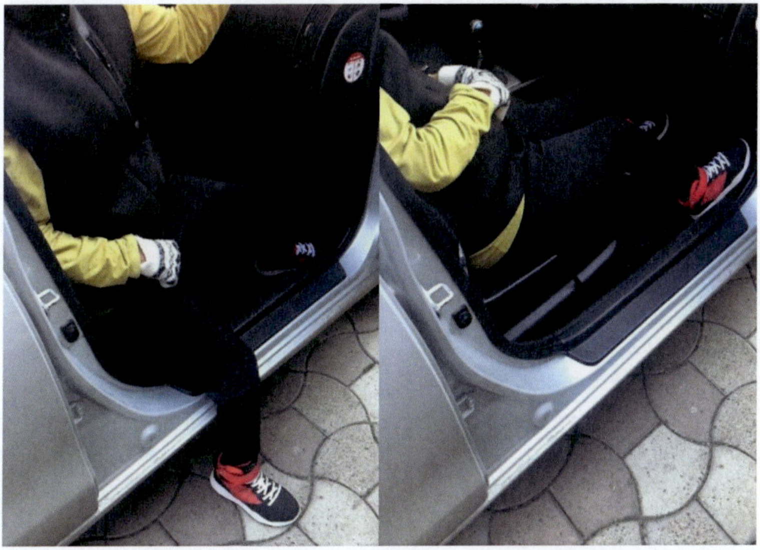

Fig. 11.20. This picture shows how an individual grabs my left leg and bends it before placing it in the car. Following the placement of the first leg in the car, the individual performs the same maneuver with the other leg. © Bianca Wiersema. Reproduced with permission from the author.

In the second method, I start by sitting on the edge of the car seat, with my feet on the ground while grabbing something fixed with my hand in order to make sure I am stable. Following that, the individual climbs into the backseat from the opposite side of the car, and grabs my forearms, as previously mentioned. After that, the individual pulls me into the car until my knees hit the seat and then places my legs in the car as explained before.

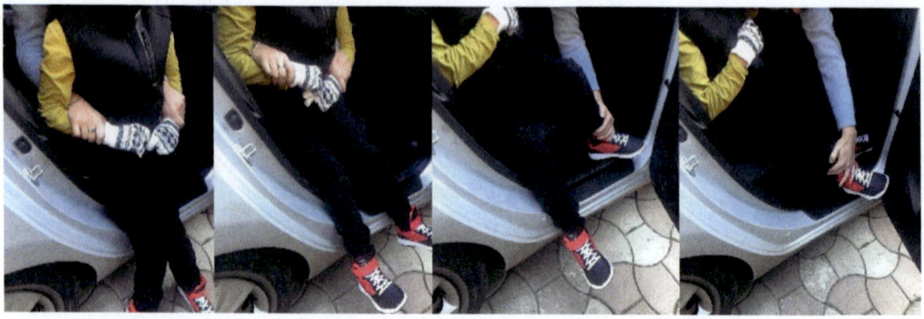

Fig. 11.21. This picture shows how an individual climbs into the backseat from the opposite side of the car, and grabs my forearms, as previously mentioned. After that, the individual pulls me into the car until my knees hit the seat and then places my legs as explained in Fig.11.20. © Bianca Wiersema. Reproduced with permission from the author.

CHAPTER 12

WALKING AIDS

Throughout my life, I have used various devices to help me walk, which I will briefly describe along with the effects I have had with each one.

a) Walking stick made of wood – in general, when I used this tool, I leaned heavily on the hand with which I held the walking stick, which led to increased spasticity, causing me a lot of pain after the effort. I leaned with my whole body on that side, not having a proper body position while walking. The wood caused my hand to slip and drop the walking stick (Fig. 12.1).

b) Walking stick with three points of support – although this one has more stability due to the three points of support, I had the same issues as with the wooden walking stick (Fig.12.1.).

c) Crutches – when using the crutches (Fig.12.1.) I tended to lean heavily on my hands, especially on my elbows, and I often lost my balance. I frequently had a lot of pain in my arm, forearm, biceps, and triceps (they became very tense and as a result, the pain increased in those areas). Too much pain in these muscles contributes to increased muscle spasticity, which can make the movement of the arm much more difficult. Pain can also occur in the trapezius muscle, particularly if you lean a lot while you walk, placing all of your weight in your hands rather than your legs. When walking with a frame with or without wheels, these issues may also arise.

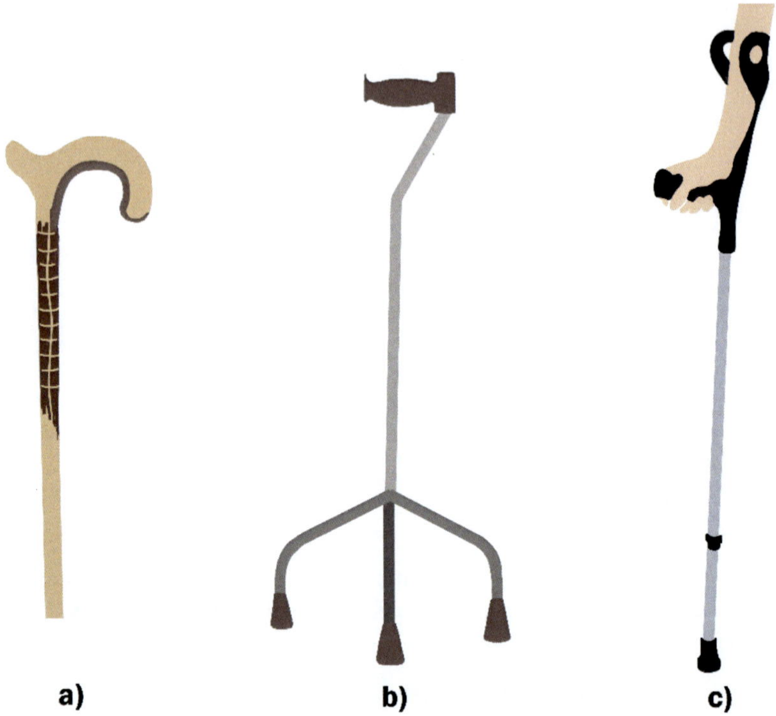

Fig. 12.1. This picture depicts (a) a walking stick made of wood, (b) a walking stick with three points of support, and (c) crutches (adapted from Baston din lemn, derby, n.d.; adapted from Echpamenteortopedice, n.d.; Forearm Crutches (Pair) - Lightweight Arm Cuff Crutch - Adjustable, Ergonomic, Heavy Duty for Standard and Tall Adults, n.d.).

➢ Walking stand with wheels (Fig. 12.2.) – despite walking straighter than with crutches or a walking stick, I was still leaning heavily on my hands while walking (which led to an increase in spasticity in the arm, biceps, triceps, and trapezius muscles). Another problem encountered was that this stand has brakes that must be used to prevent the frame from moving. A person diagnosed with spastic tetraparesis cannot make or perform two movements simultaneously since the brain can only give one order at a time. So when using the frame, the person will either walk by pushing the stand or use his hands to brake. Plainly said, the person is unable to brake while walking. If he tries, the imbalance will make him fall in front or on his back. When it comes to falling, the person tends to fall like a "boulder" or "like an airplane," because the body goes into shock and no longer responds to what is happening and becomes too spastic to allow him to move when taken by surprise. To be able to brake, a fairly large force is required in the hands, and repeated use of the brake can lead to an increase in spasticity in the hands.

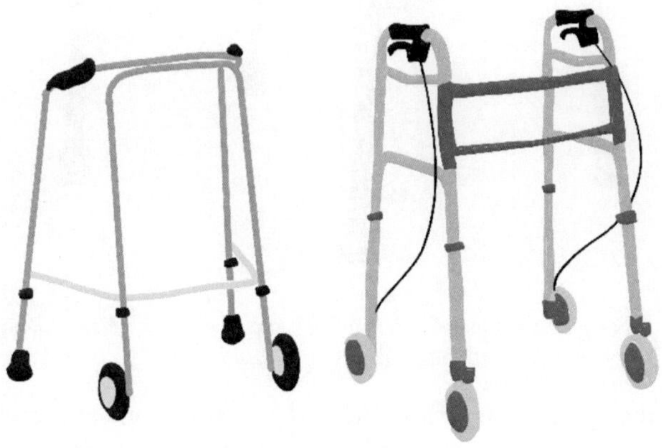

Fig. 12.2. This picture depicts a walking stand with wheels (adapted from Cadru de mers cu rotile, n.d; Cadru de mers pliabil cu 4 roti si frana , n.d.).

- Walking stand without wheels (Fig. 12.3.) – this stand is more stable because it has no wheels. Pain in the arms, biceps, triceps, and trapezius muscles may occur, as with the other devices, but it is the safest and least painful option. For me, this was the only option.

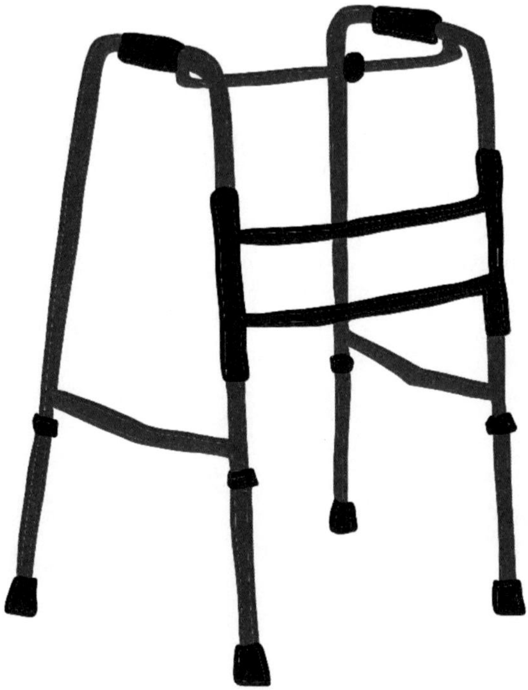

Fig. 12.3. This picture illustrates a walking stand without wheels (adapted from Cadru de Mers Fix, Reglabil, n.d.-b).

In all of the devices mentioned, the person leans a lot while walking and puts all of his weight in his hands rather than his feet. You can use this option instead of walking incorrectly with a device or if you cannot afford a fixed frame. In a flat space, sit in front of the person, who should be sitting on the edge of the bed or on a chair with his feet on the ground, take his hands, and ask him to stand up by pushing himself to his feet. If the person does not understand what it means to push himself to his feet, show the person how to do it and maybe he will understand what you are asking him and have more courage to try it. Then, make sure the person is balanced (i.e., that the person's body is upright, looking straight ahead, and that the body does not move left or right). Next, begin moving in the following manner: at each step backwards of yours, the person must step forward with the foot opposite to your foot. For example, if you step backwards with your left foot, the person must step forward with his right foot. While stepping with one foot, the person should shift his weight to the other leg on the floor, i.e., if the person lifts his right foot off the floor, the person will need to support his weight on his left foot. Perform a few daily shifts of this type to improve his mobility and balance, while ensuring that the person walks in an upright position. If he is not walking straight, remind him (even if it is exhausting) to do so.

CHAPTER 13

CLOTHING AND FOOTWEAR

Getting dressed has always been a challenge for me due to my body's limited mobility and stiffness, so I have come up with some creative ways to dress, which are listed below:

For the lower limbs

In order to wear tights or trousers, they must be elastic enough to allow them to be put on more easily. If the person has one leg more affected than the other, I would suggest starting with it because it is stiffer, and you will need more freedom in dressing it. Otherwise, you will pull the leg in an attempt to dress the other leg, causing yourself pain, which will lead to increased spasticity of the leg and thus more stiffness.

Longer trousers are preferable to short trousers because they keep you warmer. People tend to have colder legs due to slower blood circulation. Regarding tracksuit trousers or jeans, they should be a little wider and more elastic to dress the person more easily. Personally, I prefer high-waisted trousers because they keep my lumbar area warm. I recommend wool or ski trousers to keep your lower body warm. Such trousers are made for the weather pattern that you are experiencing.

There are stoppers, such as the one in Fig. 13.1., to make it easier for you to tighten the trousers yourself. Instead of making bow ties (which can be difficult to make because it requires coordination and dexterity of the hands and fingers), these can be worn on the trousers' laces. This method, however, assumes that you can grasp the stopper with your hand.

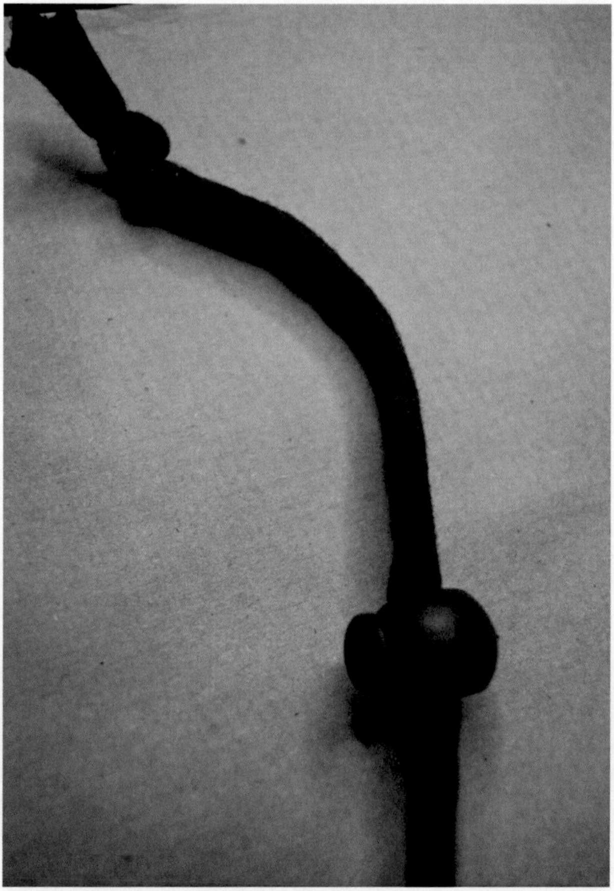

Fig. 13.1. This picture illustrates an example of a stopper to help to tighten trousers.

I tried wearing leggings, but they did not keep me warm even when I wore thick socks because they did not cover the foot.

When it came to socks, I found that the following choices worked best for me:

- ➢ Adjustable battery-powered socks that keep your feet warm for the current outdoor temperature (Fig.13.2.).

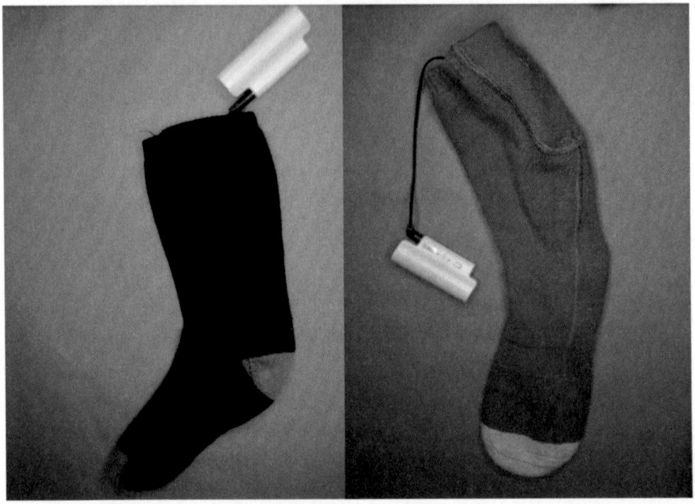

Fig. 13.2.This image shows adjustable battery-powered socks.

- ➢ Knee-high socks – they help keep the feet and legs warm.
- ➢ I also tried anti-slip socks to prevent slipping, but I got stuck to the floor (especially on the tiles) and could not unglue myself, but feel free to try them.

Heated trousers can be handy, especially when you want to keep your entire lower body warm (Fig.13.4.).

To keep my feet warm, I also use warm patches or a leg warmer (Fig. 13.5 on the upper left corner and Fig.13.7.), which work well. Also, the warm patches are available for the hands and the back (Fig.13.5. and Fig.13.6.). They should not be applied directly on the skin.

I also use an electric pillow (40x30 cm in size) to warm up my entire belly area (Fig.13.3.) and reduce spasticity there. The warm patches only heat a small area, whereas the pillow heats a larger one.

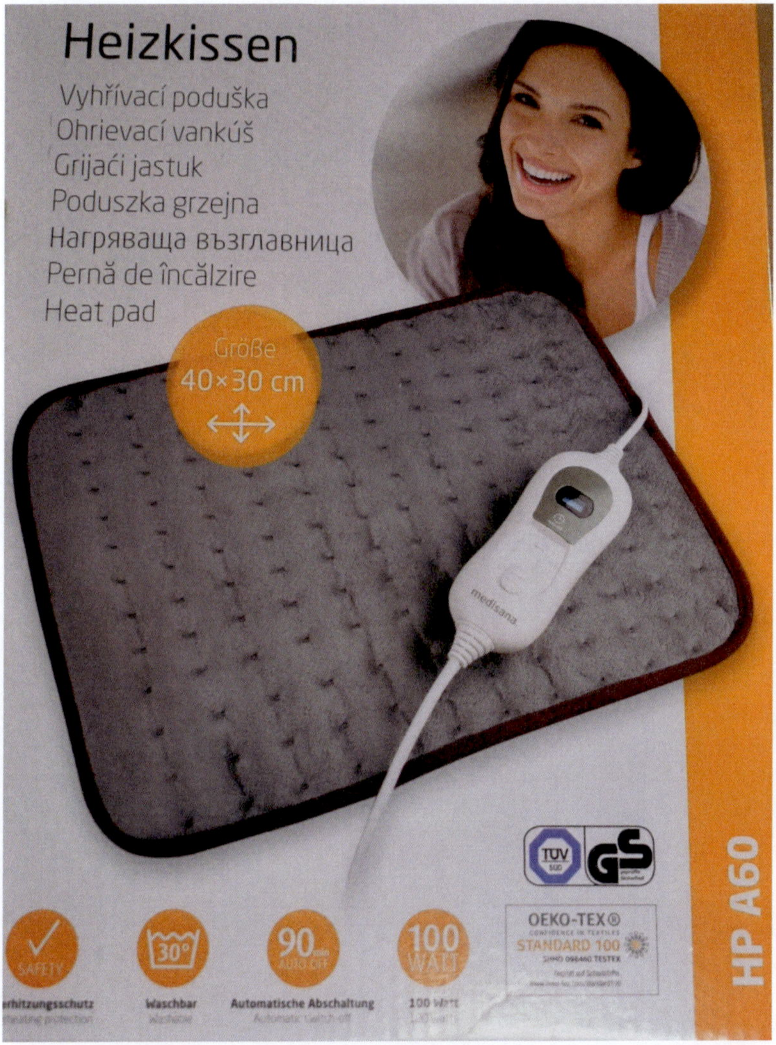

Fig. 13.3. This picture depicts an example of an electric pillow.

Skirts and dresses should be avoided because they become shorter when sitting in a chair. Due to spasticity, the legs move apart and you are unable to keep them together; this is an unintentional movement.

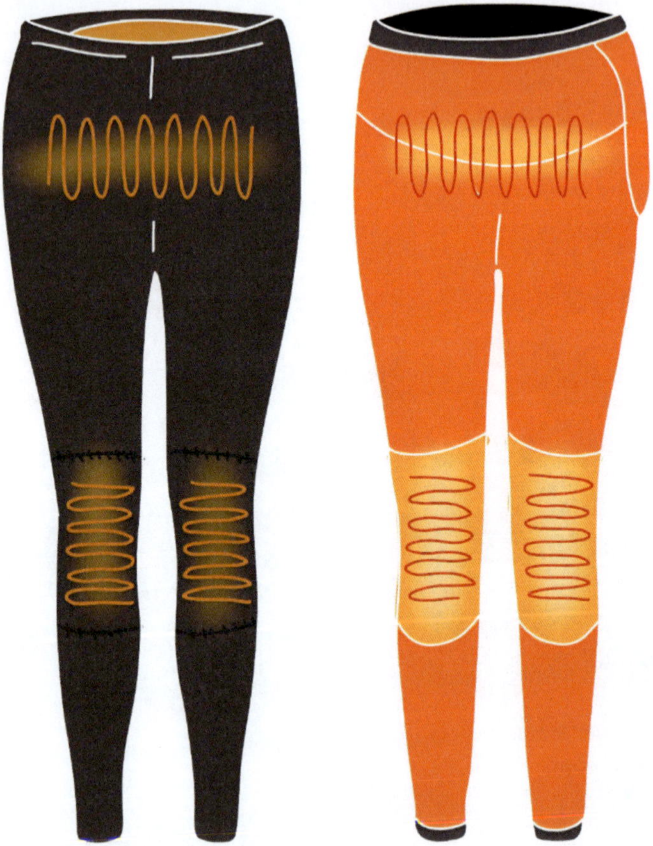

Fig. 13.4. This picture illustrates an example of heated trousers. The area heated is marked with fibre heating wires (adapted from Amazon, n.d.).

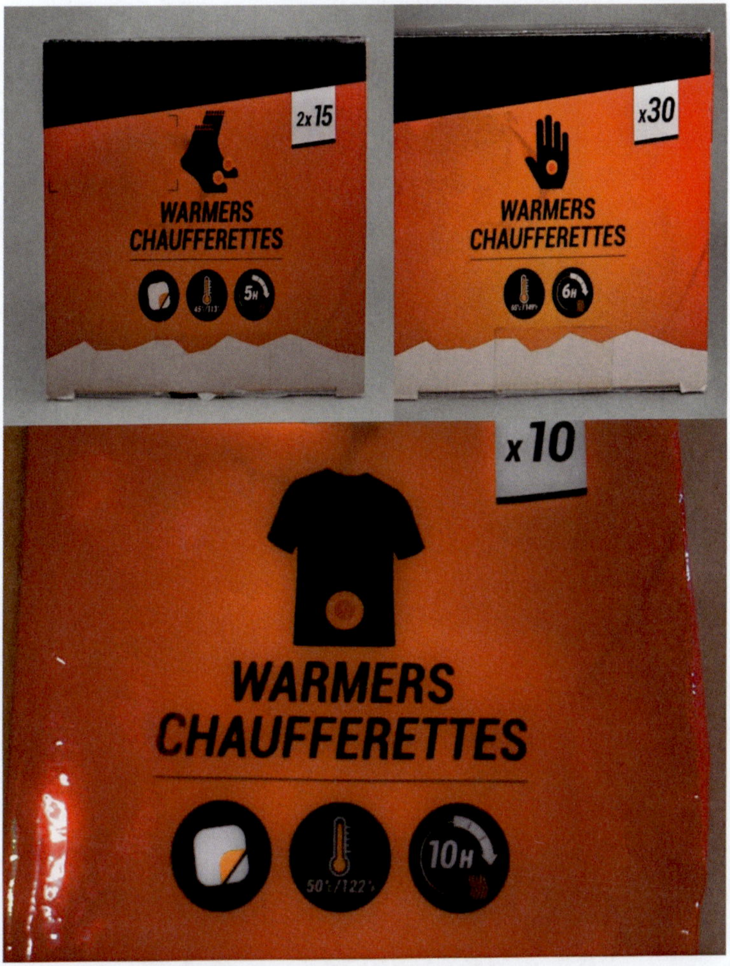

Fig. 13.5. This picture shows an example of heat patches for feet, hands and back.

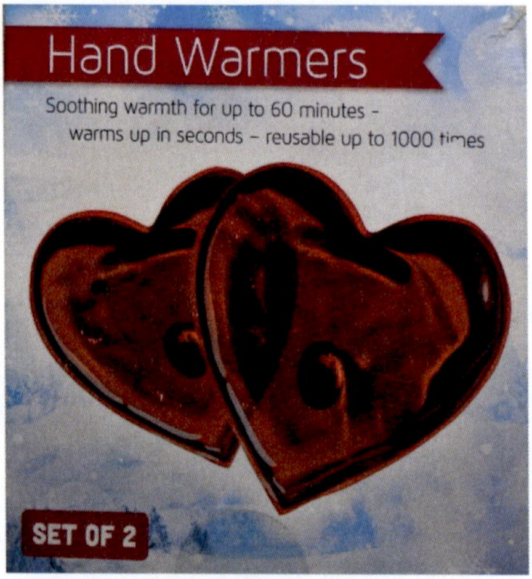

Fig. 13.6. This picture illustrates hand warmers.

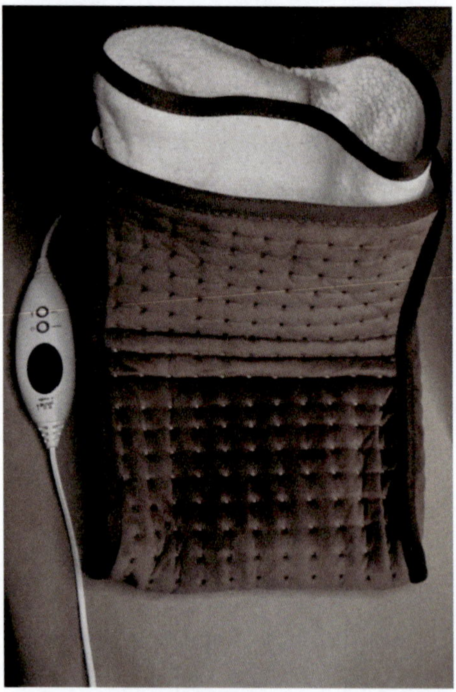

Fig. 13.7. This picture shows a leg warmer.

When it comes to shoes, the heels must be changed whenever you change your shoes or size. In general, I wear trainers that cover and protect the ankle because they provide more stability when walking and hold both the ankle and the leg in place (Fig. 13.8.).

Additionally, the heels need to be altered to fit the style of the shoes you are wearing (one type of heel suits a trainer, but not a boot).

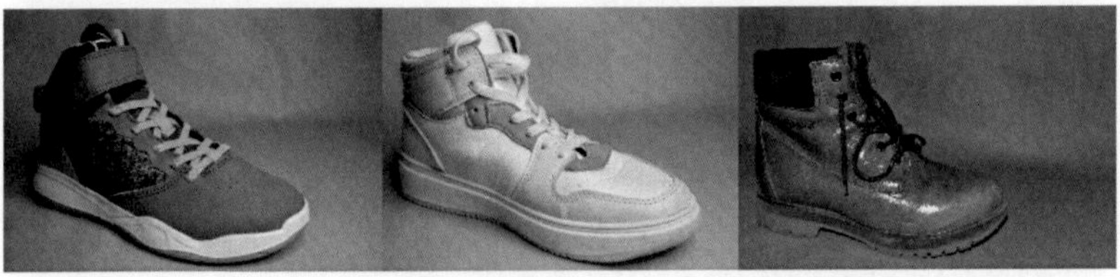

Fig. 13.8. Different types of shoes, which cover the ankle of the foot.

Regarding shoe size, I always wear a size larger in trainers or in summer shoes and two sizes larger in boots because I wear thicker socks in the winter and thus I need more space so that my shoes will not feel too tight around my feet. My feet need to slip forward a little for me to be able to walk in shoes and keep my balance. To make the shoes easier to put on and take off, I use elastic laces (Fig.13.9.). Avoid buying shoes with platforms or heels, regardless of how low or high they are, they disrupt the body's equilibrium and increase spasticity in the legs, making standing and walking difficult and painful.

Sandals can be worn as long as you do not walk in them. As there is no ankle support, it would make walking very difficult and you could lose your balance. This is the reason why shoes that cover the ankle are better in order to support the feet.

When somebody puts on my shoes I maintain a downward foot position, pushing the shoe on while rotating it left and right.

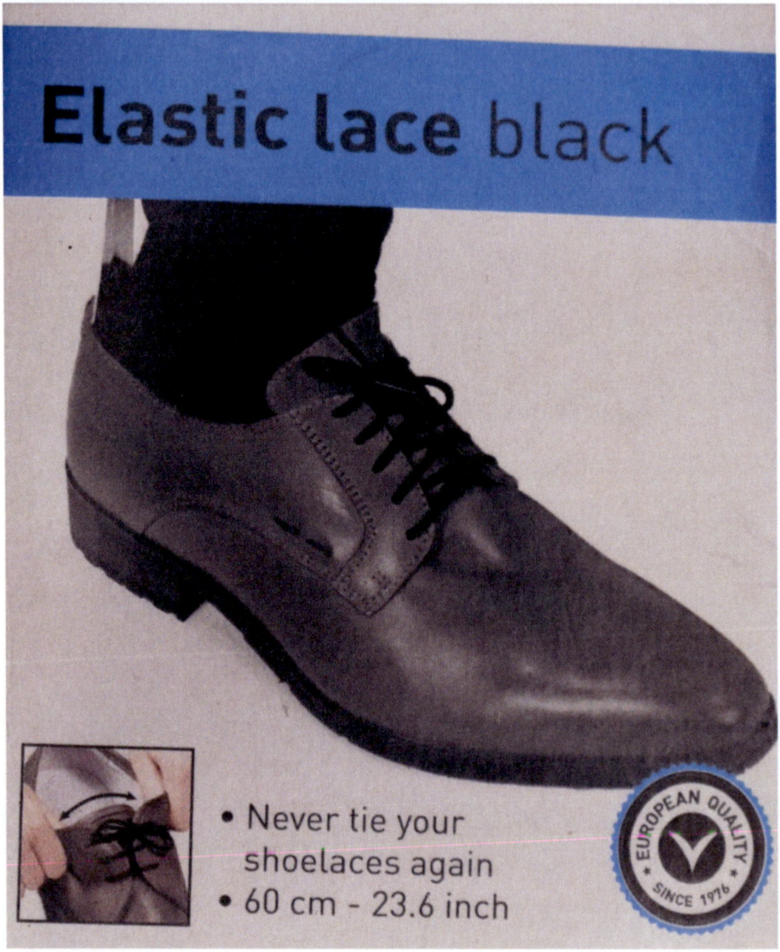

Fig.13.9. This picture illustrates an example of elastic shoelaces.

For the upper body

Blouses, like trousers, should be more elastic and wider to make dressing easier. Start with the more rigid part of the body, since that part has less mobility than the other, to prevent pain and difficulty in dressing; some people tend to dress their hands first, then their heads, while others prefer to start with their heads first, then their hands. It is entirely up to you to determine how to proceed.

Personally, I prefer stapled shirts over buttoned shirts because they are easier to button. When dressing a person in a blouse, jacket, or shirt, first make a fist in the hand and then grip the sleeve firmly in the palm to prevent the sleeve from slipping up and injuring the person's fingers (Fig. 13.10.).

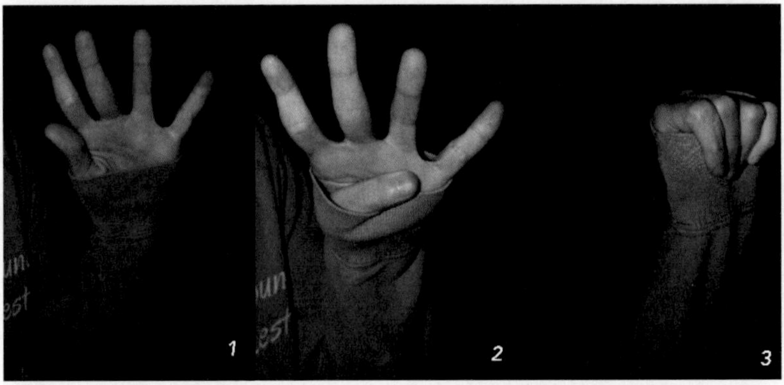

Fig. 13.10. This picture illustrates how to keep the sleeve in the hand.

Furthermore, because I am cold, I tried a heated vest with an external battery to warm my upper body. It was such a pleasant experience! If you would like to warm up your entire upper body, you can try to wear a heated vest (Fig. 13.11).

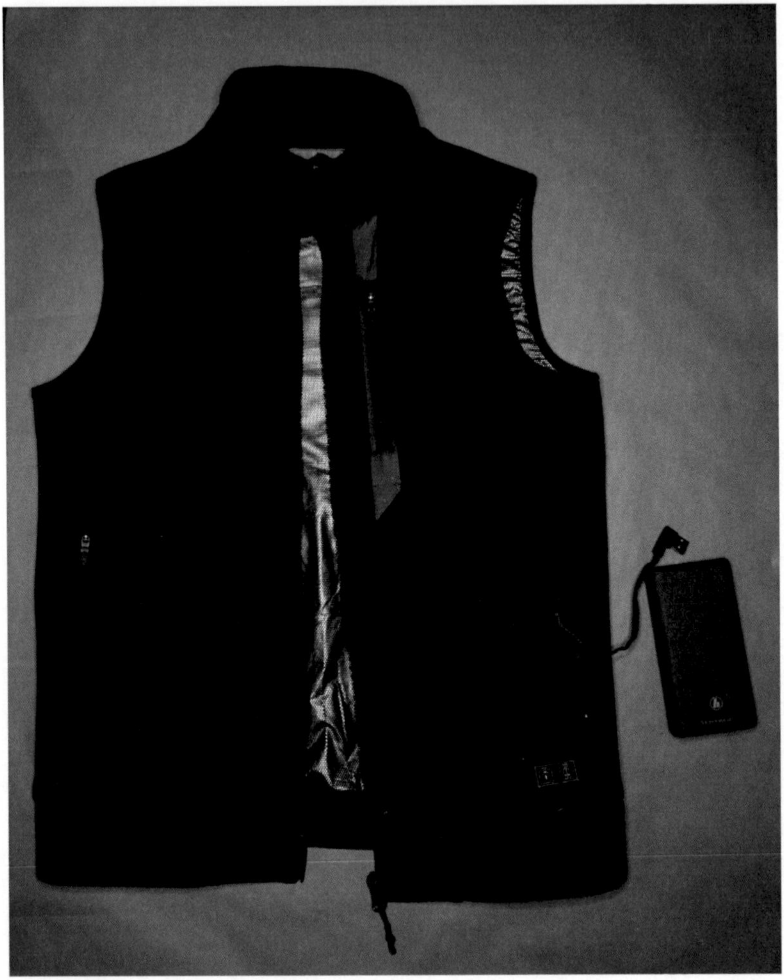

Fig. 13.11. This picture depicts a heated vest.

In terms of jackets, I prefer waterproof, windproof, and easy-to-wear jackets like in Fig. 13.12. They are comfortable and keep you warm. I wear jackets that are a size larger than my own to make it easier for me to put them on (if the jacket is too tight, dressing in it will be very difficult). Besides being water- and windproof they should also have many pockets – for practical reasons!

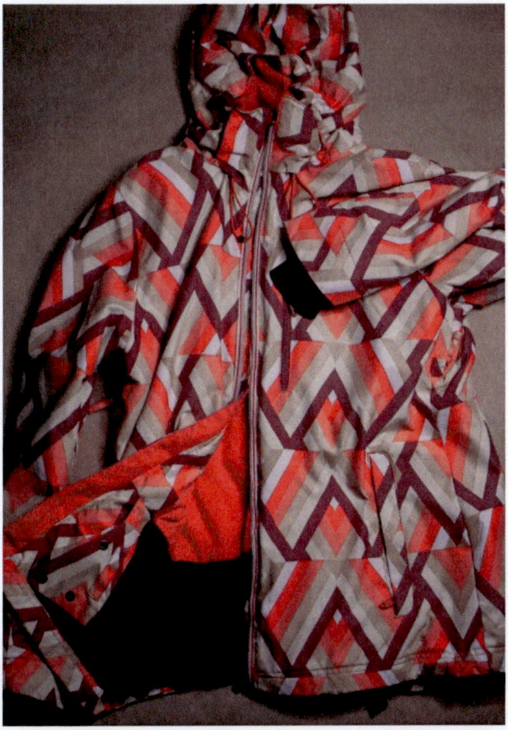

Fig. 13.12. This picture illustrates a waterproof, windproof, and easy-to-wear jacket.

CHAPTER 14

THE STUNNING DIFFERENCE A HOUSE CAN MAKE

Over the years, my family and I attempted to modify the house, particularly the bathroom, so that I could care for myself as independently as possible, based on ideas that we gleaned from the various homes and bathrooms we saw and tried in the various places we visited. The following are examples and explanations of the changes that helped me become a more self-sufficient person.

There are a few things you can do inside the house to make your life easier. It is preferable to have a non-slip floor (if not throughout the house, at least in the bathroom), with no small rugs or tiles because the person can get stuck on the carpets and can slip on the tiles.

I must always wear shoes because I cannot walk in my socks without tripping over carpets or other surfaces.

- When it comes to the bathroom, a walk-in shower with no thresholds will be the most convenient way to get in and out. A shower is preferable to a bath because it is easier to lift up the person from a chair than from a bathtub. Furthermore, the person can slip in the bathtub even if he is sitting on an anti-slip shower mat.
- A person with spastic tetraparesis cannot wash in the bathtub unless one of his parents is present to keep him in a stable position because he may have difficulty sitting alone. I could not sit alone in the bathtub because the water and my spastic muscles make me float, making it impossible for me to sit on my bottom. That is why I needed support from behind or someone to push me toward the edge of the bathtub. Also, the child can be washed in the bathtub until he is about 7-8 years old because, after that age, the person becomes more and more difficult to lift and thus it becomes more difficult to put him in and take him out of the bathtub. In order to have support on all sides and not slip, it is a good idea to have an anti-slip seat with a back and arms in the shower (Fig. 14.1.). The easiest way for

me to use the shower is to use a mobile shower head (Fig.14.2.), but the choice is tailored to the person's abilities. It is preferable to have someone check the water temperature before showering and use a protective thermostat crane to regulate the water temperature, because when the water is too cold or too hot for a longer period of time, the person feels it later, putting him at a higher risk of overheating or hypothermia (only if the person stays a longer time in cold water).

➢ If the person can wash himself, I recommend taking a mobile shower head and a shower brush (Fig.14.3.) with a long and light tail, and avoid shower sponges because they slip out of hand much easier.

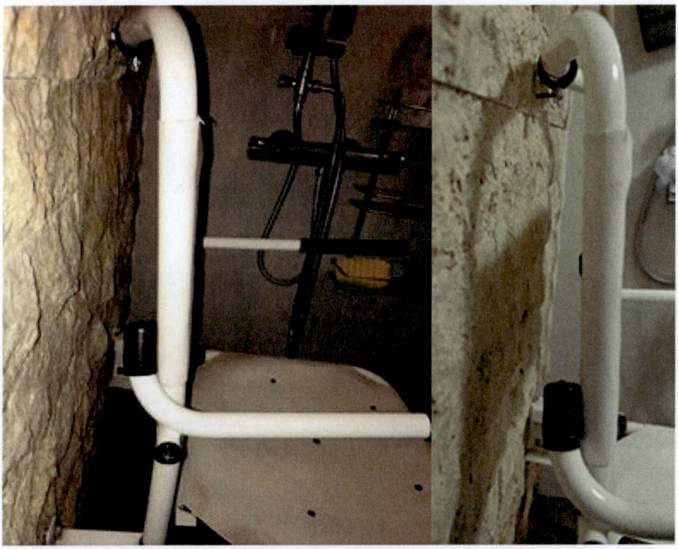

Fig.14.1. This picture illustrates a shower chair.

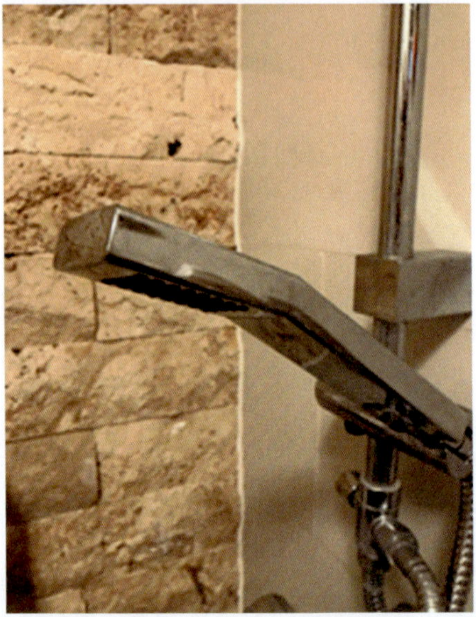

Fig. 14.2. This picture shows a shower head.

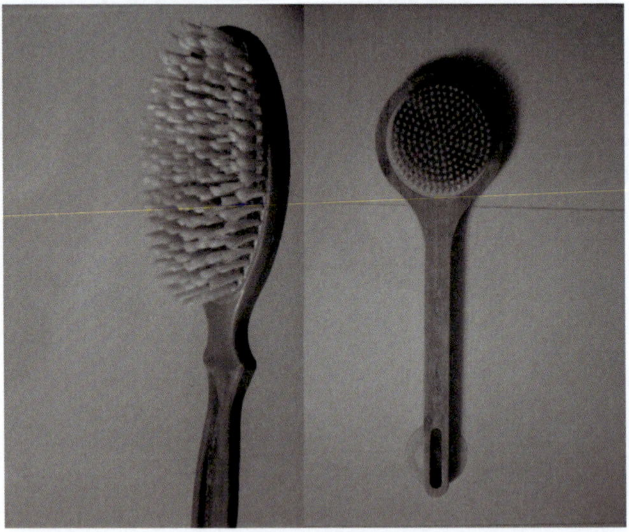

Fig. 14.3. This picture illustrates a shower brush.

- It is recommended that you have hand support on both sides of the toilet in order to maintain your balance while using it (Fig.14.4).

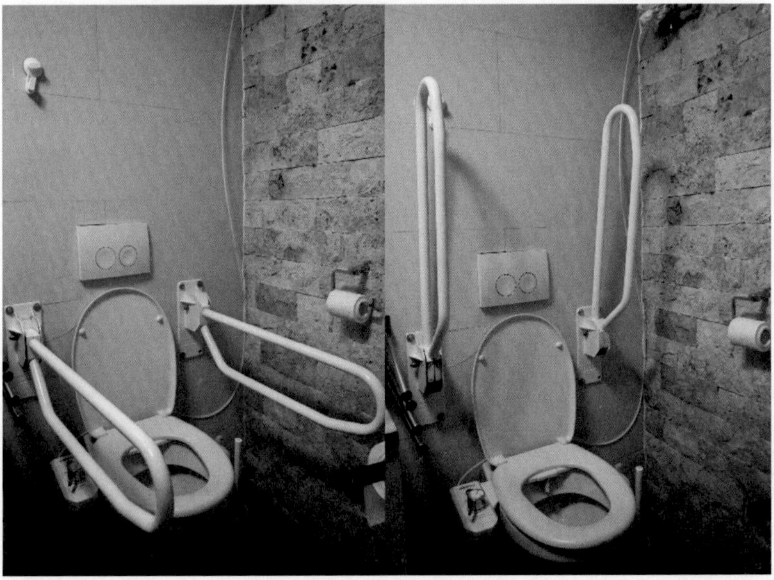

Fig. 14.4. This picture shows a toilet with hand support on both sides.

- I chose a sink with a side support to lean on and an open front (Fig. 14.5.) to make washing my hands easier (avoid oval or square sinks because the person cannot support himself with his hands, but the type of sink must be customized to the person's needs).

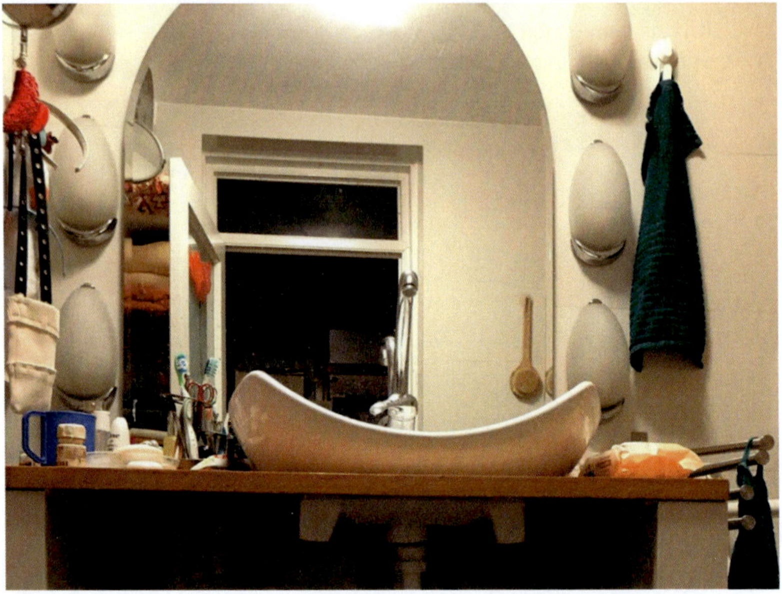

Fig. 14.5. This picture illustrates a sink with side support and an open front.

In the bathroom, I find it easier to grasp goods that are close together, but there should be enough room for you to move around comfortably. I can go from the sink to the toilet and to the shower on my own with the setup (Fig.14.6).

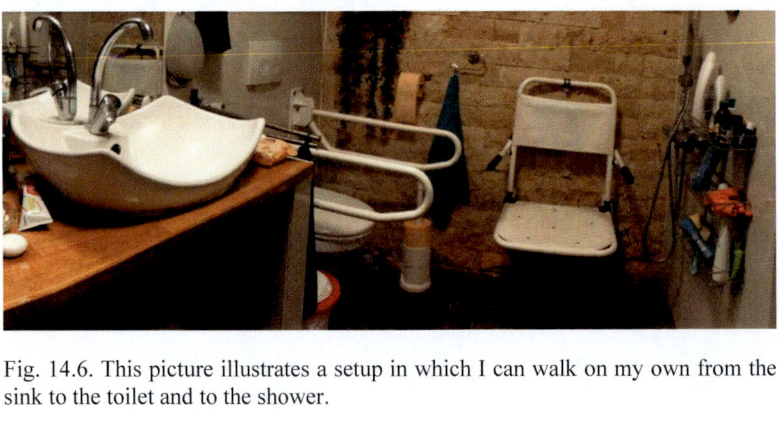

Fig. 14.6. This picture illustrates a setup in which I can walk on my own from the sink to the toilet and to the shower.

- A sensory light, which turns on and off when it detects movement in the bathroom, will also be helpful. Thus, going in and out of the bathroom will become easier too.
- Try using a hair dryer that can be turned on by pressing an on-off button, as shown in Fig.14.7. Hair dryers that can only be switched on if your finger is constantly on the button or that have a button that must be turned are impractical because they require the user to have enough strength in his hand to hold the hairdryer and make a simultaneous movement to keep the hairdryer on.

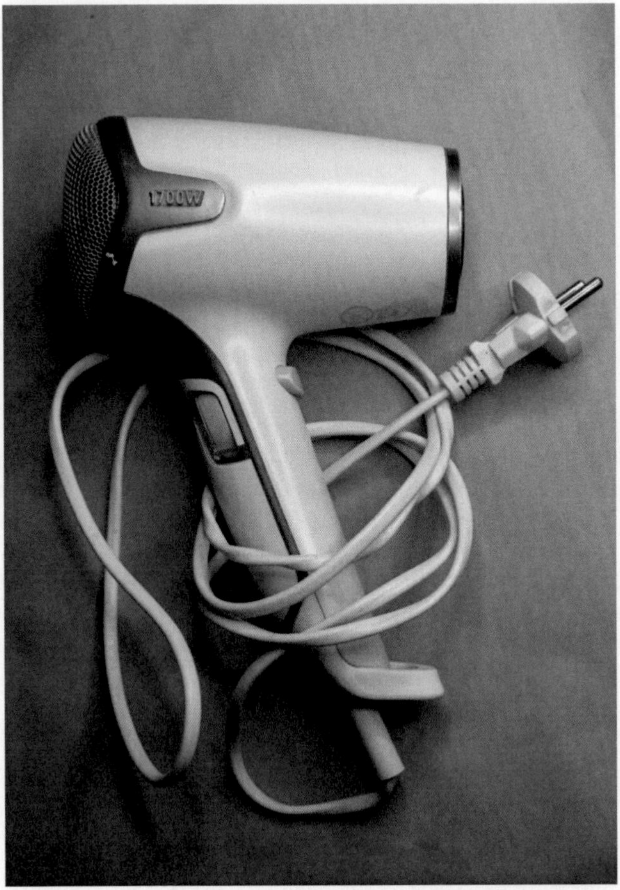

Fig.14.7. This picture illustrates a hairdryer that can be turned on by pressing an on-off button.

- Sensory trash bins can also be useful for making it easier to open and close.
- I wear shower slippers with soft rubber on the shoe sole to avoid slipping while showering.

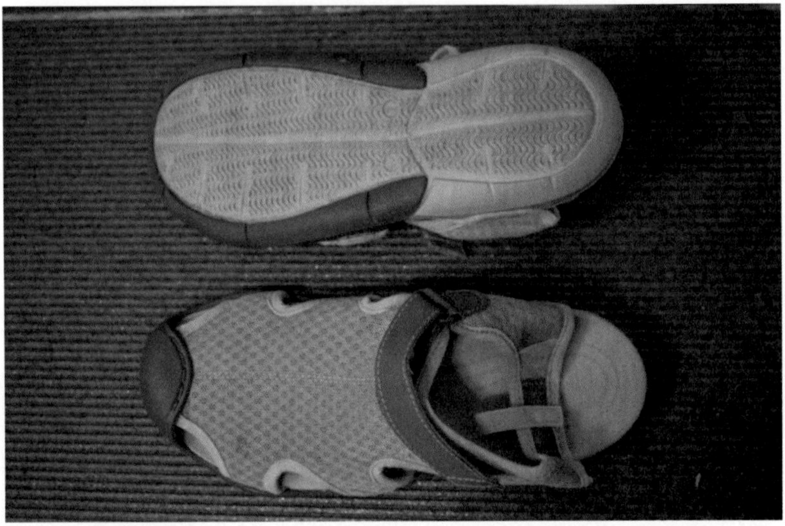

Fig.14.8. This picture shows shower slippers.

- Floor heating is a method of heating rooms that involves placing heaters directly beneath the floor. This ensures a relatively uniform heat release. Floor heating implies that the entire surface on which this system is installed is at the same level. There are two types of floor heating: water heating is accomplished through the use of pipes installed under the floor that transport hot water from the central heating system; electric heating is accomplished through the use of underfloor heating cables (Karabay, Arıcı, and Sandık, 2013, 471; Fontana 2011, 1549). The advantage of this type of heating is that your feet can stay warm all the time as the floor is always hot, which can lead to a decrease in leg spasticity and less frequent cystitis.
- In terms of turning on and off lights in the house, the easiest way would be a system that turns on the lights at the command of a voice (i.e., Alexa, Honeywell Wi-Fi Smart Thermostat With Voice Control, Ivee Sleek). Personally, I have the lighting system connected to a remote control (Fig. 14.9.). In addition, I have a

dimmable lamp next to the bed that turns on or off by touching the lower part of the lamp (Fig.14.10.).

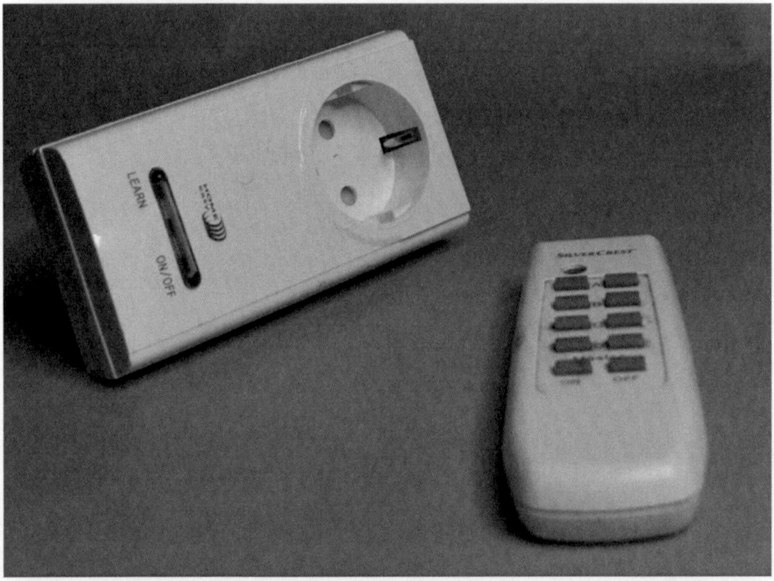

Fig. 14.9. This picture shows a system to turn the light on and off by using a remote control.

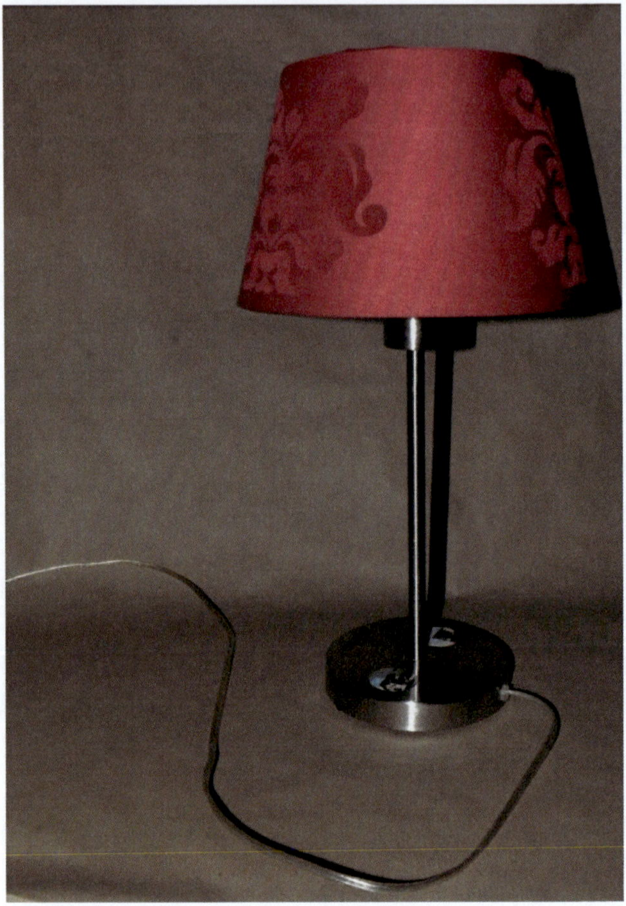

Fig. 14.10. This picture illustrates a dimmable lamp.

- The desk should be adjustable to your specific needs. To prevent from falling, keep everything in the house at the same level and avoid using thresholds. To avoid slipping while walking on the rug, I recommend rugs with a short pile rather than a longer and fluffier one.

A ramp at the front door benefits both the person in the wheelchair and the individual pushing the wheelchair because pushing the wheelchair on the ramp is much easier and the person no longer feels the shock of the stairs through the wheelchair.

CHAPTER 15

INDEPENDENCE IN THE HOUSEHOLD AND RECREATIONAL ACTIVITIES

Depending on the person's mobility, try to involve him in a variety of activities to help him develop his independence. First, you have to let the person move as much as he can, by himself with walking stands, with support, by walking with somebody, with bars, or with anything you can afford.

Teach the person to eat and drink on his own if his body mobility allows (Fig. 15.1.). I prefer hard plastic plates and cups because they are lighter and easier to handle and it gives me the possibility to do as much as I can by myself and not be helped.

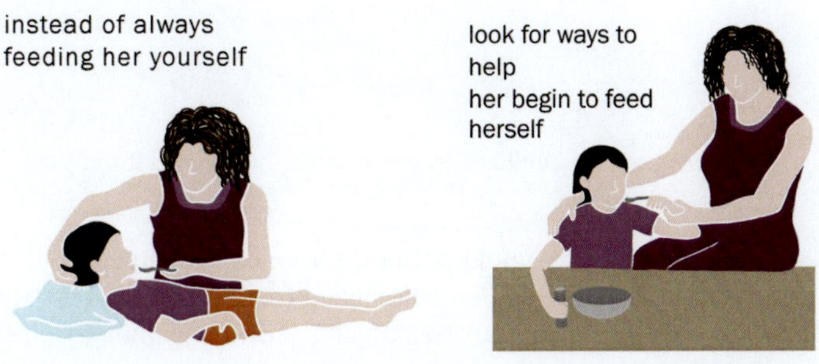
instead of always
feeding her yourself
look for ways to
help
her begin to feed
herself

Fig. 15.1. This picture illustrates how to teach a child to eat by himself (Werner, 1987, chap. 9).

If the child's head always turns to the same side, do not lie him down so that he has to turn his head to that side to see the action. Instead, lie him in a way that he must turn his head to the opposite side to see the action (Fig. 15.2.).

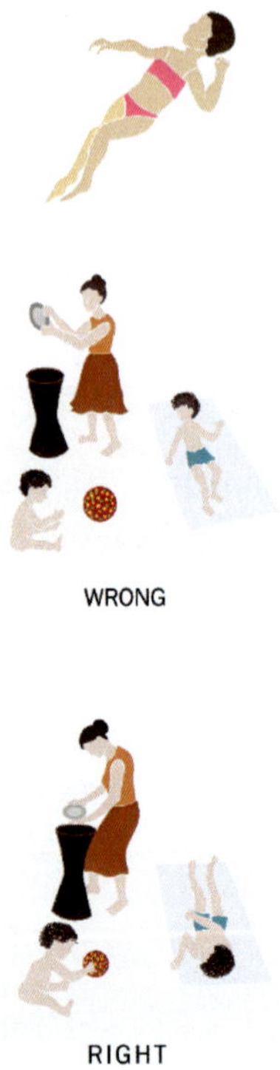

Fig. 15.2. How to position a child to lay down correctly (adapted from Werner, 1987, chap. 9).

Do not leave a child in a single position for an extended period of time as his body may gradually stiffen into that position. Attempt to shift his position on a regular basis. Alternatively, encourage him to change it. Chairs, seats, and other aids must not prevent him from moving if he can change his own position effectively (Werner, 1987, chap. 9).

I prefer to use large plastic cups because they are easier to pick up and hold (Fig.15.3.).

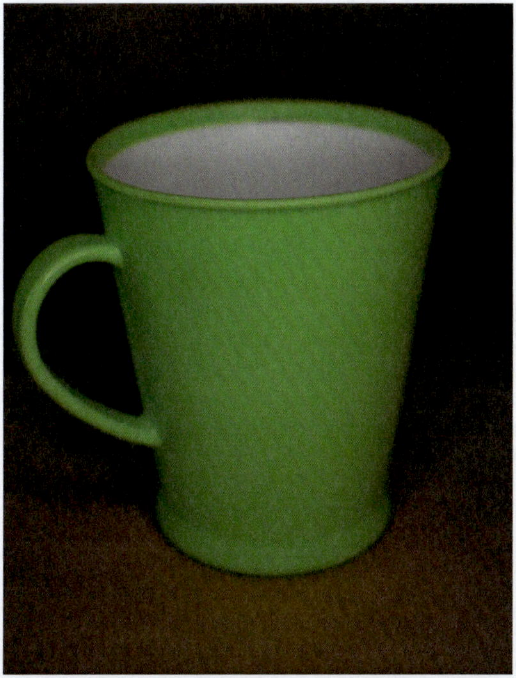

Fig. 15.3. A plastic cup with a large handle.

Fill a glass halfway with liquid rather than filling it up completely to avoid spilling the liquid when the person grabs the glass. When the glass is oval, it is more difficult for me to grasp it, so I drink with a straw, which also reduces the effort to suck. I also like using cups with handles because I can avoid using a straw.

It is preferable to avoid using thin plastic bottles in favour of thicker ones because the liquid will spill over if the person squeezes the bottle too hard. I also prefer knives that are sharp and short, which is very important, not a normal long knife. It is easier for me to cut with a shorter one. It should also have a plastic (anti-slip) grip so that it does not slip out of my hand. Allow the person to assist you in nurturing the flowers or plants if you have them in the house (for example, to tear the withered leaves) or in the kitchen cutting soft-boiled vegetables, or fresh vegetables like cucumbers, mixing a sauce, or any kind of help the person can do with his hands. Any movement is good, but do not overdo it because you become more spastic!

Personally, I can cut vegetables for the “Boeuf salad” and the Wellington. These are special dishes we make for for Christmas. I prepare them with my father every year. I can mix the cheese and eggs for the pie. I can help my parents with various things.

Try to avoid giving the person the task of peeling the shell from a boiled egg because he may grab the egg too hard (involuntarily) and break it. It is also a good idea not to let him touch hot plates because he can burn without realizing it due to diminished sensation. When something is too cold or too hot, the person feels the sensation later, so he is at a higher risk of burning himself, or when the temperatures are very low, the body freezes before the person feels that his body has frozen.

If you want to lift a person from a chair, what has usually worked for me is to pull one leg on the side of the chair, and then immediately pull the other leg so that the person sits on the side of the chair. Now you can start lifting the person by holding his hands, while the person stands on his feet in order to get up, and if this is not possible, pick up the person as done so far.

To clean my ears without injuring myself, as earpicks enter too deep, I use baby earpicks (Fig.15.4.) so I know how deep to go. If the person is unable to use the earpicks, the caregiver may use them. However, when cleaning the ears, it is best to support the person’s head so that it does not tend to move while cleaning the ears.

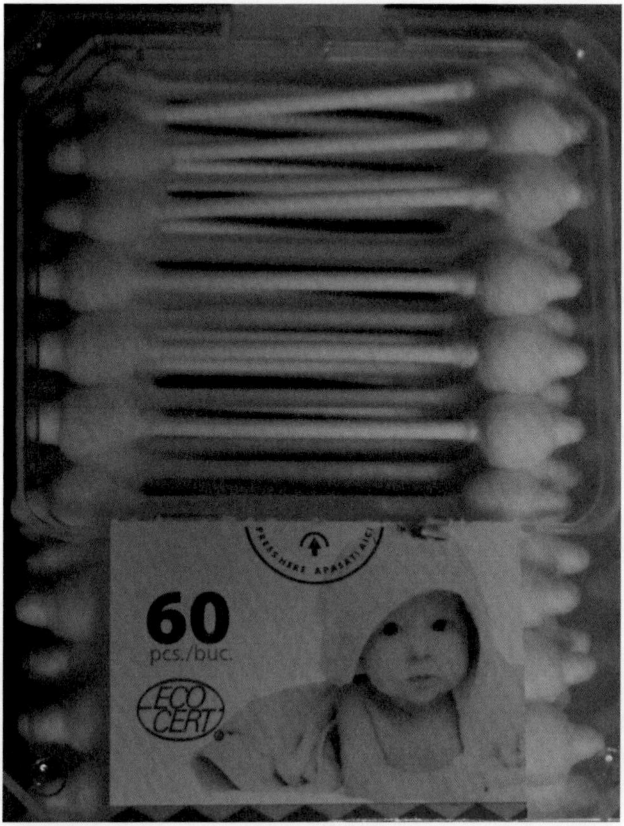

Fig. 15.4. This image depicts baby ear picks.

If the person wears hearing aids of any kind, I recommend cleaning your ears first thing in the morning before putting on your devices because the wax from the ears will shorten the life of the hearing aids. To put it in another way, the cleaner your ears are the longer your hearing aids will last. Of course, in addition to cleaning your ears, you must also clean your hearing aids periodically – how and with what please ask the otologist who recommended your hearing devices.

When there is too much noise, especially in large crowds or with lots of people, I cannot hear, and everything becomes just background noise to me.

These people need detailed explanations of the movement they have to make to help the brain process the action that needs to be done because the connection between the brain and the muscles is different compared to a healthy individual.

It may also be beneficial for someone to show the movements that should be done in order to undertake a specific action when verbalizing the movement. Visual support and a demonstration before performing it are very useful for the person who has to make that movement because he will better understand what you are asking him to do and will not panic when he has to perform it by himself. I recommend patience when explaining and demonstrating the movements, and that you give the person enough time to learn them.

Practising sport is good for the body's mobility (along with many other physical benefits) as well as the mental state of the person. Swimming is a sport that I enjoy. My body floats when I swim due to spasticity. To breathe, I put my head in and out of the water while swimming. This might tension the neck, increasing its spasticity causing pain in the affected area.

Because it can cause an increase in body spasticity, I recommend that after swimming sessions to do some physiotherapy to reduce body spasticity. For me, physiotherapy in the water did not help, but it may work for someone else.

The pool's edge must be without a lip so that the person does not hit his back when entering and exiting the water (Fig.15.5.). For the same reason, the water must reach the pool's edge. The person cannot get in or out of the pool alone; someone must help him get into the water, and when he gets out, an individual must pull up the person by the shoulders until the person is on his bottom on the edge of the pool, while another individual grabs the person's legs and pushes the person up at the same time in a coordinated manner.

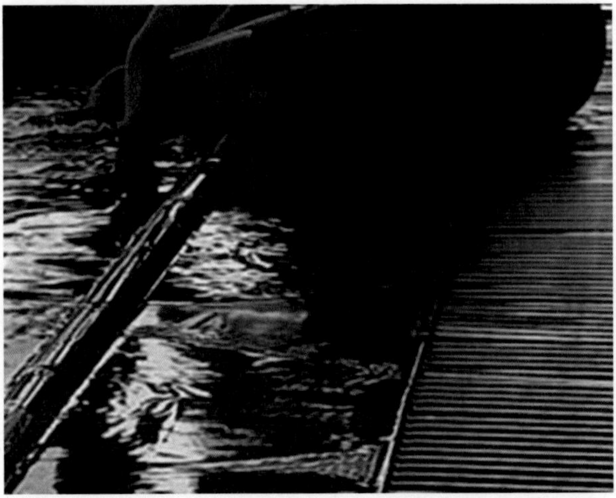

Fig. 15.5. This image shows the pool edge without lip. © Bianca Wiersema. Reproduced with permission from the author.

Sand, especially if it contains stones or is very hot, can promote spasticity in the feet.

When getting into the water, I recommend that the water temperature be at least 33 degrees Celsius in order to avoid muscle contractions caused by low water temperatures, which can increase spasticity and pain throughout the body. In some cases, especially in the summer, due to very high-temperature differences (i.e., the outside temperature is 35 degrees Celsius and the water temperature is 29 degrees Celsius), the person may go into a physical shock and start screaming due to the pain he feels. In this case, do not force the person. Instead, remove him from the water and dry him. In response to the cold, at first, a person may begin shaking uncontrollably with all limbs. Do not be scared, and keep drying him; as he warms up he will stop shaking. Make sure that the person breathes normally during this time because he may have difficulty breathing during such shocks.

When I walk near a pool, I wear anti-slip shower slippers to protect my toes and feet from injury because the pool floor is wet and I can easily slip.

Another activity that can improve manual dexterity and spatial orientation is Wire Form Maze, Montessori Pyramid and the Jenga game (Fig.15.6., Fig. 15.7., Fig. 15.8.). These games emphasise not only coordinated weight gripping, but also anticipating the movements that must be performed, which improves eye-hand coordination. Making puzzles, lego, or rubik bricks also help to improve eye-hand coordination.

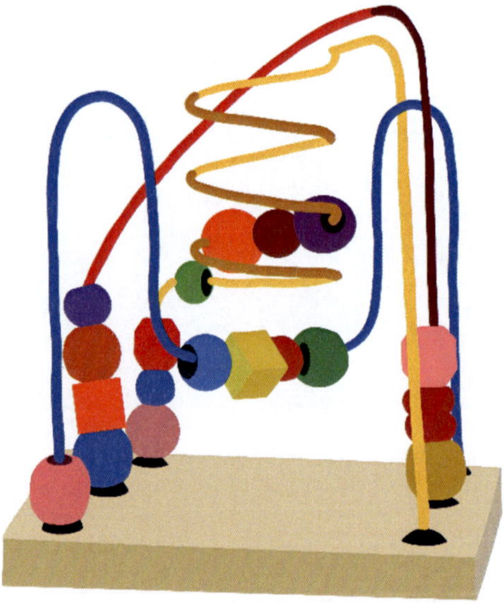

Fig.15.6. Motor Wire Forms Maze (adapted from Zorii Andrii, 2019).

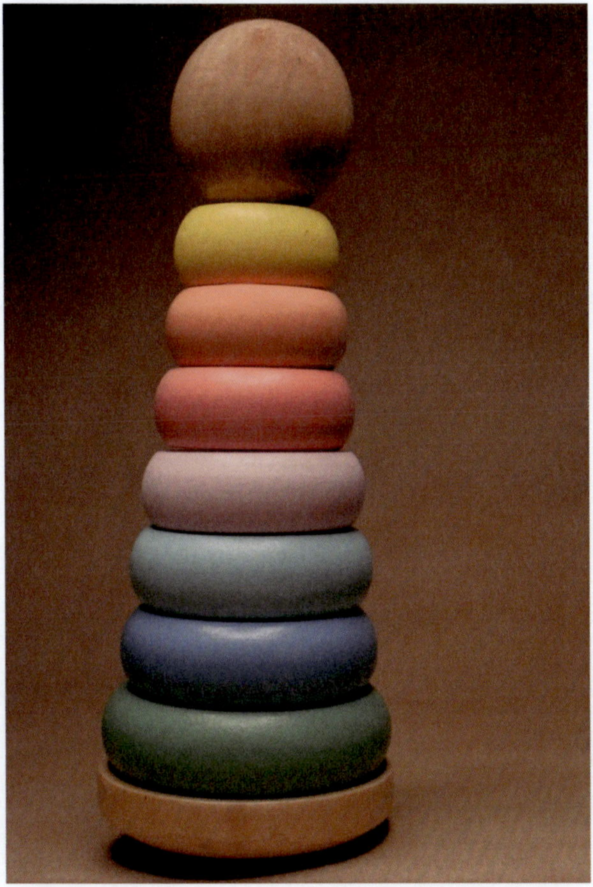

Fig. 15.7. Montessori Pyramid.

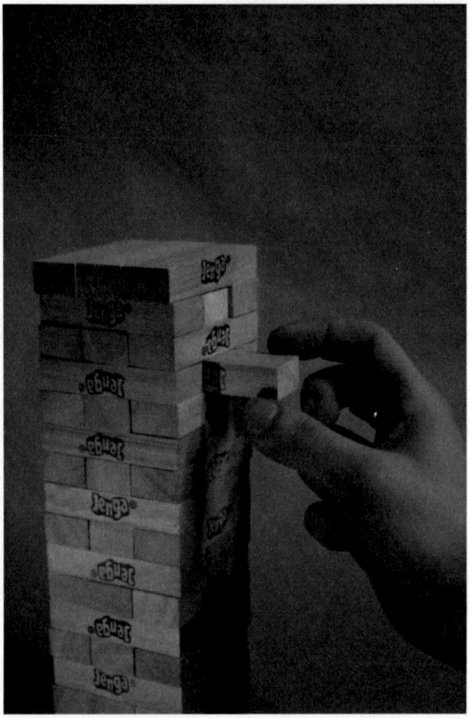

Fig. 15.8. Jenga Game.

Due to its length, a back scratcher can be used instead of a fork to give the person the possibility to scratch himself (Fig.15.9.).

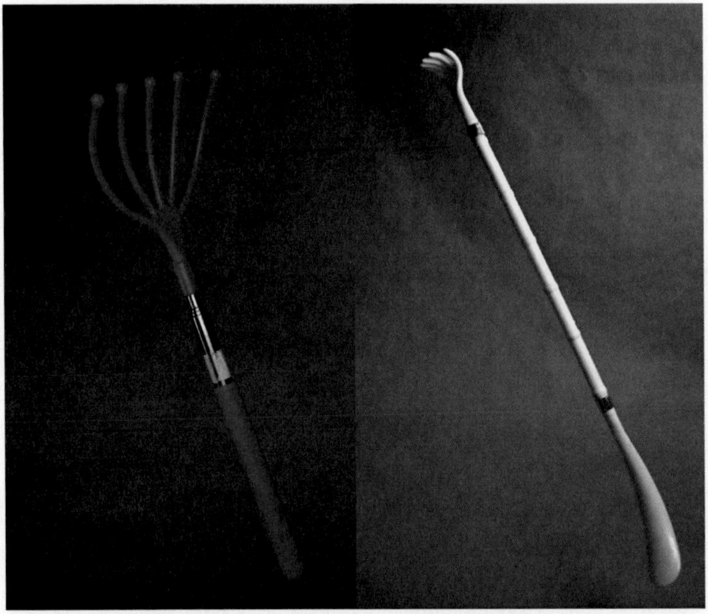

Fig. 15.9. This image illustrates two types of back scratchers.

Allow the person to dress himself if he is able (of course, at first, you have to teach him how to do so). When I put on a blouse, I start with my head, then the most affected hand, holding my fist closed to avoid hurting my fingers, and then the other hand, as described in the chapter Clothing and Footwear. Afterwards, I grab the shirt and pull it down.

It is recommended to involve the person in as many activities as possible allowing him to experiment and discover what he enjoys. Doing things on his own increases the person's self-esteem and independence. Engaging in too many activities can also lead to increased spasticity, but lack of movement will have the same effect, so I recommend you find a balance in your actions.

Whenever possible, choose skills and activities that will help the child become more independent and capable of doing more for himself and others. Do not overprotect the child in order to help him prepare for greater independence (Werner, 1987, chap. 34).

CHAPTER 16

MEDICAL TREATMENT

a. Medications and their side effects

The following are some of the medicines that have helped me manage spasms and pain. It is recommended that you should not combine them and that you seek medical advice about how many and for how long to take them. Before taking them, read the side effects and see what to expect if any arise.

- ➢ Mydocalm is a muscle relaxant that should only be used on the advice of a doctor; it should not be used for an extended period of time.
- ➢ Nurofen and/or paracetamol help to relieve pain.
- ➢ Calmogen is a supplement that will help you relax when you are feeling agitated or anxious.
- ➢ Melatonin – Use melatonin only if you are unable to sleep regularly (I used it because I could not sleep due to the pain). Try something herbal before taking melatonin (which is a chemical). It takes 20 minutes to an hour for melatonin to take effect, so use it only when absolutely necessary. Melatonin should not be taken for an extended period of time, and driving is not recommended after taking it. Valerian is a much more natural alternative to melatonin.
- ➢ Use Mentat if you need to memorize a lot of details in a short amount of time. It is natural and works very well even if taken for a longer period of time.
- ➢ Encephabol, Cerebrolysin, Tonotil-N, and Tanakan are used only on the recommendation of a neuropsychiatrist for chronic brain disorders; consult a neuropsychiatrist for indications for usage; indicated for neuronal regeneration.
- ➢ Cannabidiol (CBD), shown in Fig.16.1., helps to reduce spasticity. I used CBD (which does not contain Delta-9-tetrahydrocannabinol (THC)) only in conjunction with physiotherapy to help reduce my

spasticity. CBD on its own does not replace physiotherapy, it is only an adjuvant to assist in managing spasticity.

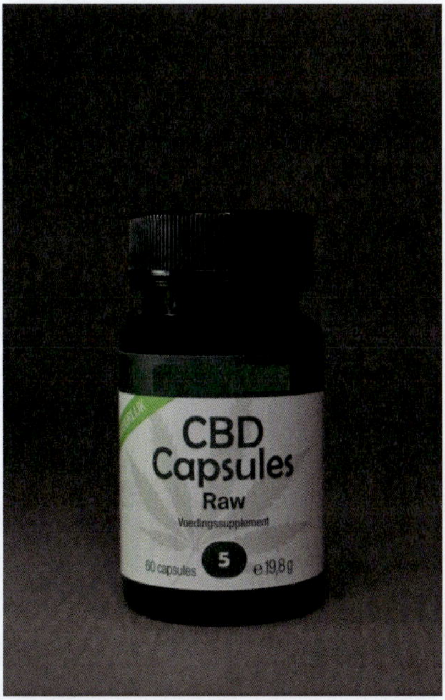

Fig.16.1. This image shows an example of CBD pills.

I used a number of different approaches to deal with constipation.

Every laxative causes dehydration, so drinking water or other liquids is necessary to prevent dehydration after taking it.

- ➢ Duphalac liquid – consult a pharmacist about the appropriate dose; read the instructions before taking the liquid and drink plenty of water afterwards to avoid dehydration.
- ➢ You can also take one sachet of Casenfibra or Macrogol per day, mixed with water or juice to make it easier to drink (Fig. 16.2.).

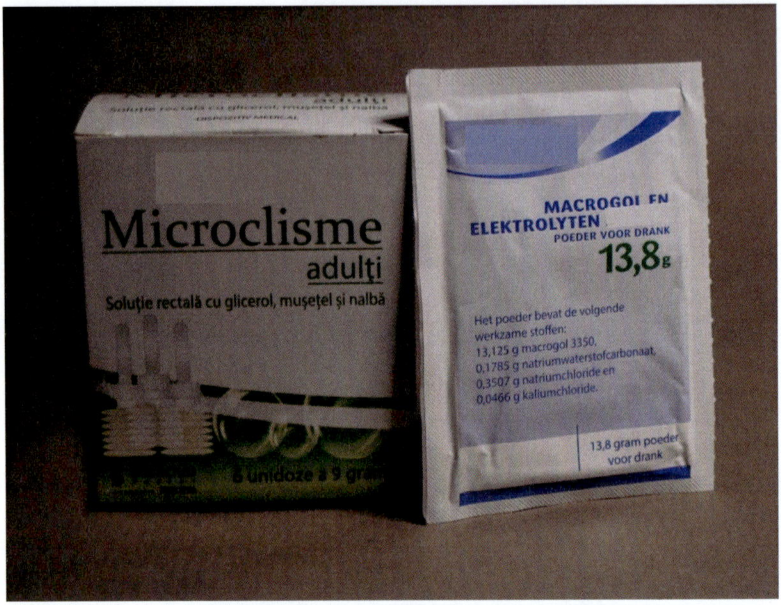

Fig. 16.2. This picture illustrates and example of Microenema and Macrogol

- If the evacuation does not occur after attempting a variety of techniques, you may use a 5 ml syringe filled with soap and water, or short plant microenema (longer ones are more painful). Vaseline, shower gel, or soap can be used to make it easier to insert the microenema or the pipe into the anus, which must be done straight rather than tilted, in order to prevent damage to the anus mucous membrane from the plastic. Use soap and shower gel only if you have no other choice because they irritate the mucous membrane of the anus.

I use Hermozon cream, which contains tetracycline and hydrocortisone acetate, for the treatment of hemorrhoids. Cortisone in high doses and for an extended period of time can cause hallucinations, sleep problems, and weight gain, among other side effects. Pilex ointment cream is a plant-based alternative to Hermozon cream.

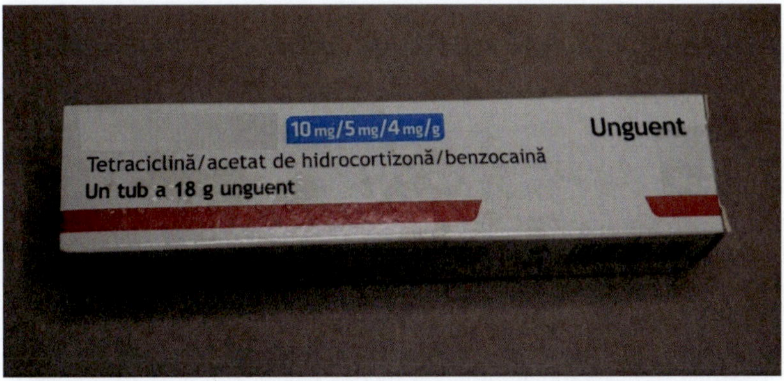

Fig. 16.3. Hermozon cream (adapted from Hemorzon unguent, n.d.)

Personally, after 4-6 weeks of taking, say, Casenfibra, the effect of evacuation has diminished because my body has become used to it, so I try to alternate between different methods.

When a pill is taken for an extended period of time, the body becomes tolerant to it and, as a result, its effectiveness diminishes. You can become easily addicted to pills, and quitting is even more difficult. When you want to stop taking the medication that you have been taking for a longer period of time, you may experience withdrawal symptoms, which might cause pain and can lead to an increase in spasticity in the body. When giving a pill to a person, try to help the person to maintain his balance by supporting the back when the person drinks water because the person may lean back his head while drinking, which can lead to loss of balance.

Check for potential side effects before taking the medication, since it is preferable to avoid symptoms than to experience them. As for me, I experienced almost all the rare side effects of most of the medications that I took.

b. Botulinum toxin

Botulinum toxin is a drug (toxin) that is administered by a specialist at a specific time to help relax muscles. It is used to treat a variety of medical conditions (Orsini et al., 2015; Jankovic, 2004), including spastic tetraparesis (Multani et al., 2019). I recommend reading the package leaflet for more information about this medication.

Although all of my doctors said there would be no side effects from my botulinum toxin injections, I experienced them all at once. The side effects I experienced are listed in Appendix B.

I would like to start by saying that after the fourth round of injections (the dosage is specified in Appendix B), I could not stand (nor keep my balance, or walk, and even a cup was too heavy to keep in my hand). Sitting was impossible because I could not keep my balance. Furthermore, I was in a state of continuous and deep sleepiness (I slept 23 hours a day and struggled a lot to stay awake for an hour), carrying out any kind of activity was impossible because I was too tired and did not know what to do with my body, I could feel all the muscles on my body burning, I had difficulty eating and swallowing food (and drinking fluids), pain in the eyes area, muscle weakness and it all culminated with severe headaches that did not subside with any medication.

A round of injections included one injection in each of the following members: right and left brachial upper limbs, right and left supinator, right and left semimembranous lower limbs, gastrocnemius 2 right and 2 left points.

The movements were more difficult to be performed because my brain was used to another movement that required different coordination, the muscle was not contracted and had to exert effort, which caused me more pain.I could not swim anymore because my muscles were not responding to my commands as a result of the botulinum toxin. As my spasticity helped me to float, my body could not float in the absence of spasticity. I could not even make active-passive movements on my own when I was doing physiotherapy. The physiotherapist performed all of the movements in a passive manner.

The most common indication for botulinum toxin type A (BoNT-A) therapy in CP is to treat focal muscle overactivity in children who can walk in order to improve gait and function (Koman et al., 1993; Cosgrove et al., 2008).

You must understand that a person who does not know or has not learned to walk before taking botulinum toxin will have no idea what to do with his body after having this medicine. Therefore, if the brain does not send the signal to perform a certain move, this person will have no way of knowing how to walk, as the botulinum toxin only relaxes the muscles and does not replace the signal to the brain.

There were 19 reported deaths following BoNT-A injection, with children being more likely to die than adults (Montastruc et al., 2016). Death and serious adverse events are rarely reported in randomised controlled trials (RCTs), highlighting the need for continuous recording and monitoring of serious adverse events in community settings (Graham et al., 2008; Montastruc et al., 2016). In Australia, at least four non-ambulant children with cerebral palsy died as a result of BoNT-A injection, with other events going unreported or underreported (Graham et al., 2008; Montastruc et al., 2016, Graham, H.K., 2019).

Over the past 15 years, a growing body of literature has described the negative effects of BoNT-A injection at the level of the injected muscle (Multani et al., 2019; Fortuna et al., 2011; Minamoto et al., 2015). The majority of reviews of BoNT-A fail to mention the dangers of muscle atrophy and fibrosis (Graham et al., 2000; Multani et al., 2019; Cocco and Albanese, 2018).

CHAPTER 17

SURGERIES

The observation of the patellar reflex is one of the clinical trials done most common for neurological tests, making it an important tool for the diagnosis of many neuromuscular diseases (Beers, M. H., 2004).

The patellar reflex is a deep tendon reflex that is mediated by spinal nerves from levels L2, L3, and L4, primarily in the root L4. The patellar reflex test is used to determine the neurological function's integrity by striking the patellar tendon below the knee cap with a test hammer (Fracois, R., 2003).

The patellar reflex happens when there is a sudden change in muscle length; in this case, the tendon is stretched as a result of the application of the hammer stroke (Tortora, Derrickson, Tzal, Gutiérrez, and Diana Klajn, 2002; Waterhouse and Campbell, 2008). A sudden leg extension must be the expected response. A diminished or heightened response is a sign of injury or disruption to the quadriceps muscle's innervation (Palmer and Epler, 2003).

Numerous conditions, ranging from tumors in the spinal cord (Mendioroz and Poza, 2003) to illnesses like the Guillain-Barre syndrome (Michelli, F., 2002) that affect the peripheral nervous system (Kelly, E. B, 2012), may alter the patellar reflex response.

Other factors that can interfere with the test result include the intensity of the stroke (Dafkin et al., 2013), the patient's nervousness during the test, and the patient's age (Chandrasekhar et al., 2013).

The goal of developing an objective quantification for the test has emerged in recent years (Dafkin et al., 2013; Lebiedowska, Siddhartha, Avinash, and Garmirian et al., 2011; Chung et al., 2015). Some research has attempted to quantify the test by performing motion analysis (Tham, Abu Osman, Wan Abas, and Lim, 2013) on children with cerebral palsy (O'Sullivan et al., 2016).

If the leg does not react to the hammer, it means that the motor information does not exist and the leg has neuronal lesions, meaning there is no neuronal signal and therefore the leg is completely paralyzed, and thus no operation will be effective because the person will never be able to walk.

When I was born, my groin legs overlapped, my knees were bent, and I began walking on tiptoe rather than on my entire foot, as shown in Fig.17.1. So, over time, I became friends with the operating room, undergoing operations that, although painful, provided me with greater mobility of movement, but this mobility was obtained in conjunction with intensive postoperative recovery. For more information about my medical history, consult Appendix A.

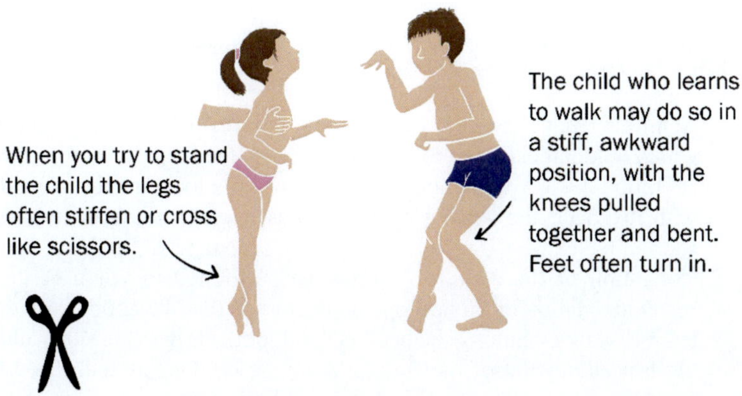

Fig. 17.1. This image depicts children who cross their legs like scissors and keep their knees bent when walking (adapted from Cerebral Palsy | Sethu, 2005).

I had several surgeries to improve my body's mobility over time, which are briefly listed below, with more information available in the Appendix A. Because total anesthesia is not recommended due to the neurological side effects, I had Rahie anesthesia in all of my surgeries.

The surgeries entailed tendon elongation as follows:

➢ To the adductors in order to keep my knees in the correct position (because I overlapped my groin legs, as shown in Fig. 17.2.). Unfortunately, the elongation of my left leg was not done properly; the tendon was cut too wide, and as a result, my leg went to the side when walking; it took me a lot of extra exercises to control my leg while walking compared to the other leg.

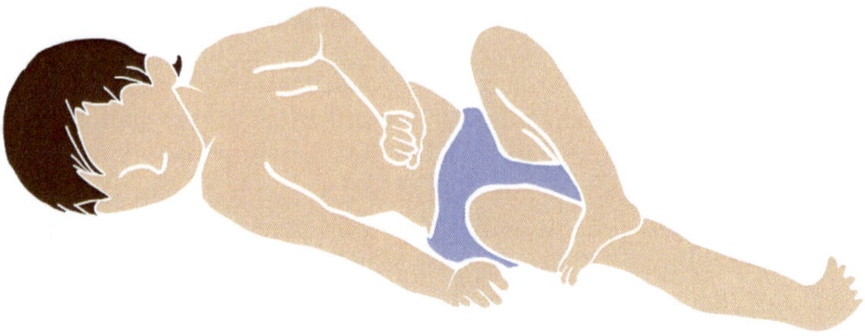

Fig. 17.2. This image shows how a child overlaps his groin legs (adapted from Hinchcliffe, 2007).

- Achille's tendon (twice) – to be able to put the heel on the ground, which automatically led to the correction of the balance (before the operation, I was walking on my tiptoes, without touching the ground with my heel; the second operation was necessary due to tendon shortening caused by body growth). I recommend that the first elongation of the Achille's tendon be performed in youth at the recommendation of the orthopedic doctor, so that the child starts to learn to walk by putting the heel on the floor as early as possible, and the last elongation of the Achille's tendon be done after the body finishes growing. It is critical, when allowed by the orthopedics doctor and physiotherapist, to start to put your foot down gradually and to learn to walk on the entire foot and not on your tiptoes.

  The elongation of the adductors was performed when I was 4 years old. My first elongation of the Achille's tendon was at 7 years old and the second, and hopefully last, at 17 years old.

- Tenotomy of the bilateral tibial-hamstring muscle in order to fully stretch the knee (before the operation I kept the knee bent, without being able to stretch it), as shown in Appendix A-Figures 1 and 2.

  Because of the pain caused by the cast in the heel area, the doctors cut a piece in that area to relieve pressure and pain as shown in Fig.17.3.

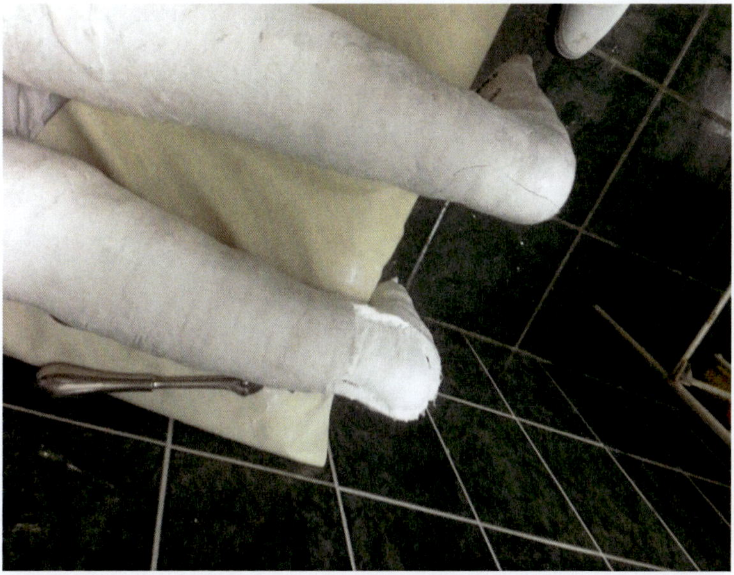

Fig.17.3. This image shows the heel area where the cast was cut. © Bianca Wiersema. Reproduced with permission from the author.

The surgeries were only performed on the advice of the primary orthopedic doctor and with the approval of the primary neurologist. In order to maximize the benefits of the surgery, it is critical to begin post-operative recovery as soon as possible. Recovery is best accomplished with the help of a physiotherapist who has postoperative recovery experience. If physiotherapy is not performed following tendon surgery, the tendon elongation caused by the surgery will be ineffective, and immobilization in bed will make everything worse.

According to David Werner (1987, chap. 9), surgery can sometimes be used to treat severe, persistent contractures. Surgery to weaken or release spastic muscles, however, is less frequently successful and occasionally worsens the situation. A thorough analysis is required. Only if the child is already walking and is having increasing difficulty due to contractures should surgery typically be considered, in order to help the child walk independently. Surgery typically will not help a child who cannot balance well enough to stand and walk by himself. Cleaning and bathing can be made easier with surgery to separate the legs.

Due to the fact that I do not walk independently, my orthopedic doctor advised that any surgery that could help me walk more easily would be ineffective. I walk only assisted by a walking aid or a person. The ones described above helped me become more independent, like bathing or walking with assistance but did not make me walk on my own.

CHAPTER 18

VACCINATIONS

Regarding vaccines, I was immunized at a young age with all of the vaccines deemed necessary at the time. I had no side effects other than the pain at the injection site.

Because the diagnosis of spastic tetraparesis can make you more vulnerable to more serious forms of other diseases, it is recommended that you get vaccinated, but only with a doctor's permission and under medical supervision.

When the COVID-19 pandemic began, I was unsure whether or not to get vaccinated because of my diagnosis. After consulting with my family doctor, I decided to do it.

I experienced pain at the injection spot, muscle weakness, and a headache for about 3 days following the initial dose. After the second dose, I felt again pain at the injection spot, insomnia (5 days), and chills (1 night). After the third dose, the injection spot hurt, I had nausea, and mild dizziness for about 2 days.

It is critical to be healthy at the time of vaccination in order for the vaccine not to attack any sickly areas of the body that you are unaware of. After all, it is preferable to be safe rather than sorry.

I also had COVID, experiencing all possible symptoms: hot flashes, chills (especially at night), headaches, dizziness, muscle pain, breathing issues, loss of taste and smell (about 4 days), stuffy nose, fatigue, and low resistance to effort for a week.

After my test came back negative, I experienced respiratory distress, fatigue, and low resistance to effort for one month and two days following the positive test.

Keep moving even if you get tired more frequently and try to maintain your mobility if you can. With the physiotherapist, go over the exercises you can and cannot do at this time. Lack of movement will lead to increased spasticity.

CHAPTER 19

BETTER SAFE THAN SORRY

There is a widespread misconception that people with disabilities cannot have a sex life, have sexual desires, or be sexually attracted to someone or all of them at the same time – an idea that is supported by no solid evidence in our society.

Sexuality manifests itself in a variety of ways and is an important part of each individual's development and life.

Although I support the contraceptive pill, it is contraindicated in certain medical conditions, including the diagnosis of spastic tetraparesis, because it can result in the following complications, which outweigh the benefits, among others (Fasen et al., 2020):

- Stroke
- Heart attack
- Thrombosis

A consultation with your family doctor and gynecologist is needed to decide which form of contraception is best for you. Do not use any form of contraception without first consulting your doctor. Depending on your desires and needs, the best option is to use contraception measures such as a condom, ring, or IUD. AND DO NOT FORGET TO ENJOY EACH OTHER!

THE CONDOM is a thin rubber sheath that wraps around a man's penis (Fig. 19.1.). During sex, it prevents the man's sperm from entering the woman's vagina and womb. Latex condoms provide the best protection against sexually transmitted infections (STIs) and HIV (Werner, 2011, chap. 20).

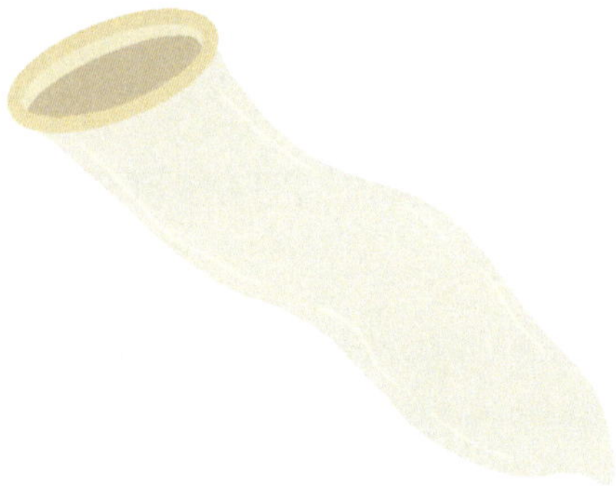

Fig. 19.1. This picture illustrates a man's condom (adapted from Werner, 2011, chap. 20).

THE WOMEN'S CONDOM is a thin, plastic sheath that fits inside the vagina (Fig.19.2). The condom is held in place by a flexible ring at the closed end. The other ring hangs out from the open end, covering the vaginal outer lips. The female condom is the most effective method of protection against pregnancy and STIs, including HIV, that is controlled by women. The female condom should not be used in conjunction with a male condom (Werner, 2011, chap. 20).

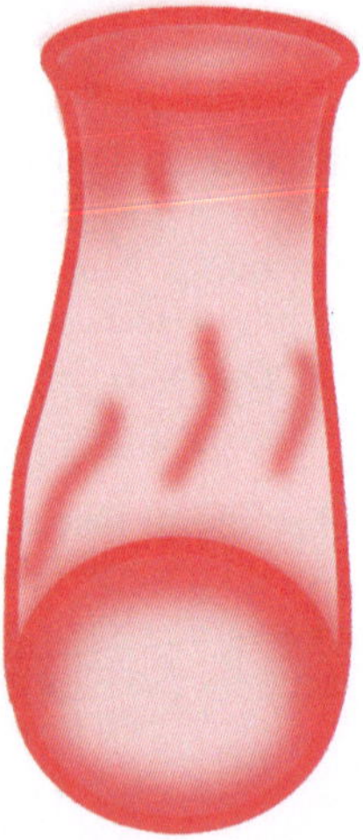

Fig. 19.2. This picture depicts a women's condom (adapted from Werner, 2011, chap. 20).

THE DIAPHRAGM is a shallow cup of soft rubber worn by a woman in her vagina (Fig. 19.3). It can be used whenever you want and should be left in for at least 6 hours after having sex. A diaphragm may provide some STI protection (Werner, 2011, chap. 20).

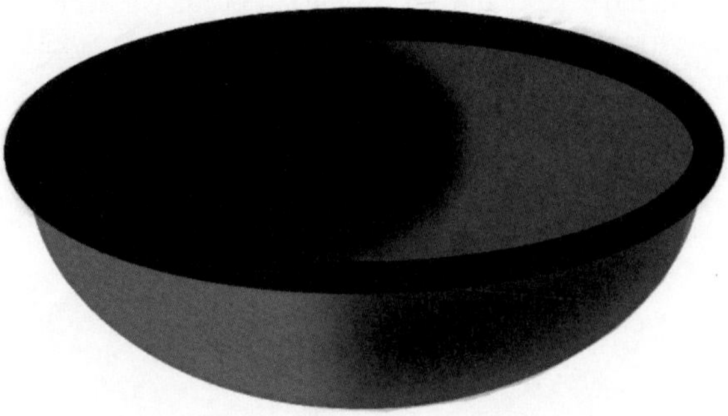

Fig. 19.3. This image depicts an example of a diaphragm (adapted from Werner, 2011, chap. 20).

SPERMICIDES are vaginal foam, tablets, cream, or jelly that are inserted before having sex (Fig. 19.4.). Spermicide destroys a man's sperm before it can enter the womb. It does not provide protection against STIs or HIV. Between 10 and 15 minutes before having sex, place a tablet in the vagina. Foam, jelly, or cream work best when applied to the vagina just before sex. Every time you have sex, add spermicide. Do not shower or wash the spermicide out for at least 6 hours after sex. Some spermicides can cause vaginal itching or irritation (Werner, 2011, chap. 20).

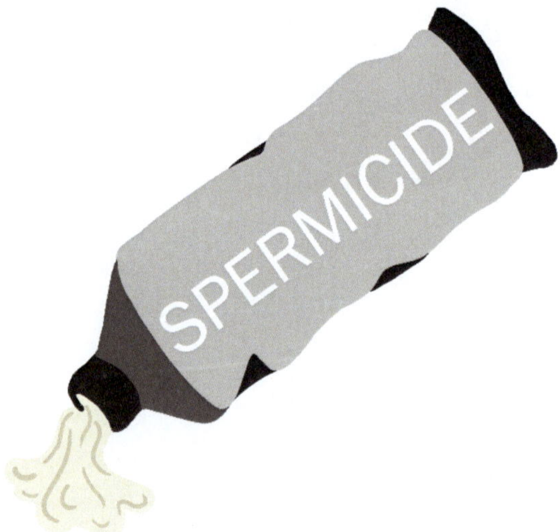

Fig. 19.4. This image shows an example of spermicide (adapted from Werner, 2011, chap. 20).

THE INTRAUTERINE DEVICE (IUD) is a small object that a specially trained health worker inserts into the womb (Fig. 19.5). The IUD prevents the sperm of the man from fertilizing the egg of the woman. The IUD can be inserted whenever a woman and her healthcare provider are reasonably certain she is not pregnant and has no signs of a vaginal infection or a STI. When a woman wants to change methods or become pregnant, she can ask a trained healthcare worker to remove the IUD. The IUD provides no protection against STIs (Werner, 2011, chap. 20).

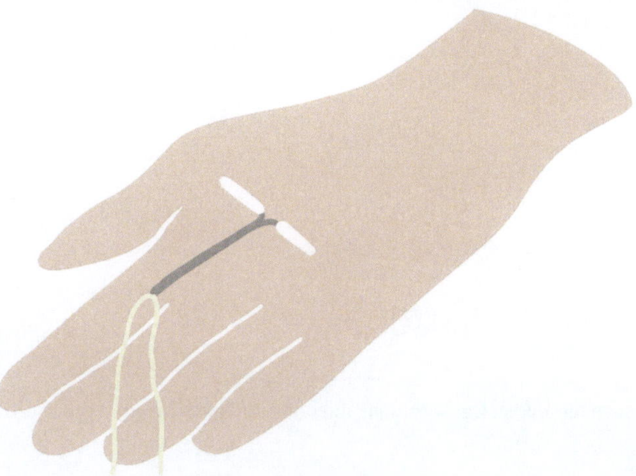

Fig.19.5. This image shows an intrauterine device (adapted from Werner, 2011, chap. 20).

INJECTIONS – hormone injections (Fig.19.6.) are given to a woman every 1 to 3 months (Werner, 2011, chap. 20).

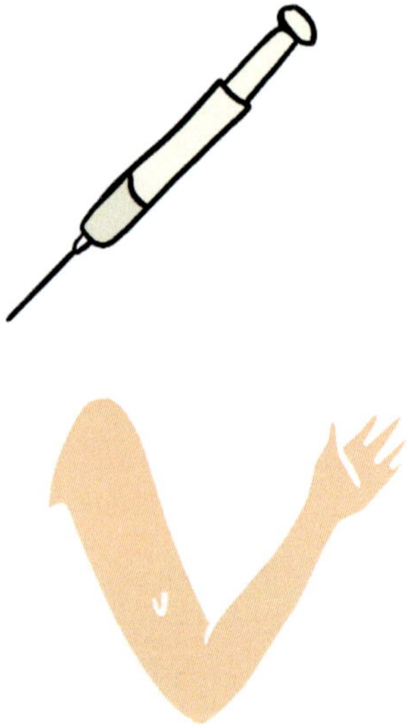

Fig. 19.6. This image depicts a hormonal injection (adapted from Werner, 2011, chap. 20).

IMPLANTS are small, soft tubes that are implanted beneath the skin of a woman's arm. Depending on the type of implant, these tubes contain the progestin hormone and can prevent pregnancy for 6 months to 5 years (Werner, 2011, chap. 20).

The use of intrauterine devices as a method of contraception is not advised because the pelvic and intrauterine muscles may be spastic as a result of the diagnosis, and the effect of these devices on spasticity is unknown.

There are hormonal contraceptive methods such as the contraceptive pill, IUDs, contraceptive implants, contraceptive injections, contraceptive plaster, and the ring. These contain hormones, which are contraindicated because they can cause complications, especially in the case of a diagnosis of spastic tetraparesis. There are also non-hormonal contraception methods such as the diaphragm, coitus interruptus (pulling out), external and internal condoms.

Many of the methods are inaccessible to people with disabilities; for example, the diaphragm cannot be used by itself nor can spermicide. Condoms, IUDs, sex without intercourse, pulling out, and sterilization are thus the safest and most feasible methods.

STERILIZATION. There are relatively safe, simple operations for both men and women who do not want to have any more children. These operations are often free in many countries. Inquire at the health center. STIs, including HIV, are not prevented by sterilization (Werner, 2011, chap. 20).

• For men, the procedure is known as a vasectomy. It is simple and quick to perform in a doctor's office or a health center, usually without putting the man to sleep. Small cuts are made here in order to cut and tie the tubes from the man's testicles (Fig.19.7.). The testicles are not removed. The procedure has no impact on the man's sexual ability or pleasure. His fluid is the same, but it contains no sperm (Werner, 2011, chap. 20).

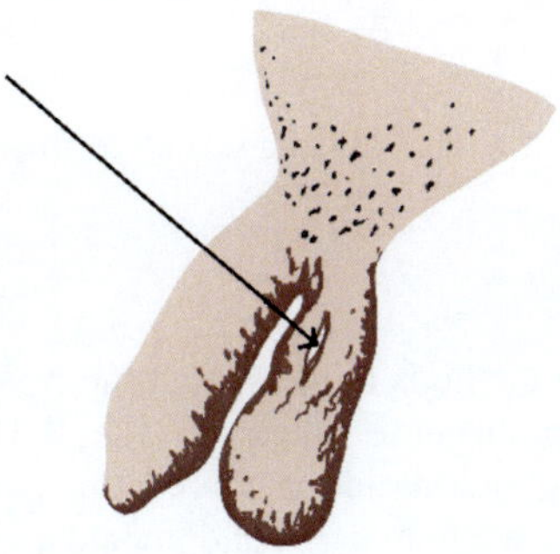

Fig. 19.7. This image shows a vasectomy procedure (adapted from Werner, 2011, chap. 20).

• For women, the procedure is known as a tubal ligation, which means "tying the tubes." A small cut is made in the lower belly and cut and tie the tubes coming from the ovaries, or egg-makers (Fig.19.8.). It is usually possible to perform it without putting the woman to sleep in a doctor's office or health center. Although the operation is usually successful, women are at a higher risk of infection than men. This procedure has no effect on a woman's menstrual cycle or sexual ability, and it may make having sex more pleasurable because she is not concerned about pregnancy (Werner, 2011, chap. 20).

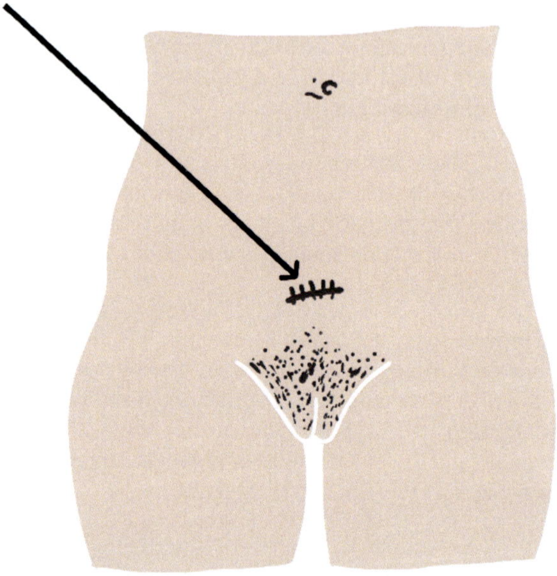

Fig. 19.8. This image depicts a tubal litigation (adapted from Werner, 2011, chap. 20).

Methods that combine

It often helps to use two methods at the same time if you want to be more certain that you will not become pregnant. The IUD combined with a condom, diaphragm, and spermicide is more effective than any of these methods alone. Similarly, if a man uses condom and a woman a diaphragm, the chances of pregnancy are lower than if only one method is used (Werner, 2011, chap. 20).

When both the man and the woman are committed to avoid pregnancy and prevent one another from STIs, methods for contraception are most effective (Werner, 2011, chap. 20).

The chart on the following page illustrates how well each contraception technique prevents pregnancy and offers STI protection. The chart's stars indicate how effectively each method prevents pregnancy (Table 19-1.). A method will function better if both a man and a woman employ it correctly each time they engage in sexual activity (Werner, 2011, chap. 20).

To put it in a nutshell

Table 19-1. Contraceptive methods (adapted from Werner, 2011, chap. 20)

Contraceptive method	Protection from pregnancy	Protection from STIs	Possible side effects	Other important information
Condom for men	★★ Good	GOOD		The condom is most effective when it is combined with spermicide and lubricant.
Condom for women	★★ Good	GOOD		When the woman is on top of the man during sex, it is less effective.
Diaphragm (with spermicide)	★★ Good	SOME		When combined with spermicide, it is most effective.
Spermicide	★ SOME	NONE	skin allergy	When combined with another method, such as a diaphragm or condom, it is more effective.
Hormonal methods Birth control pill, patch, injections Implants	★★★ Very Good ★★★★ BEST	NONE	headaches, nausea, and fluctuations in monthly bleeding	These methods may be unsafe to women who have certain health issues. Consult a health professional.

Sex without intercourse (penis not inside the vagina at all)	★★★★ BEST	SOME		Couples may struggle to adhere to this method.
Pulling out (withdrawal-coitus interruptus)	★ SOME (LOW PROTECTION AGAINST PREGNANCY)	NONE		When combined with another method, such as spermicide or diaphragm, it is more effective.
IUD	★★★★ BEST	NONE	monthly bleeding that is difficult and painful.	This method may be unsafe to women who have certain health issues. Consult a health professional.
Sterilization	★★★★ BEST	NONE		After this procedure, neither men nor women will be able to have children.

CHAPTER 20

WHAT YOU SHOULD AVOID AND WHY

Throughout my experiences, I have tried a variety of methods to increase my independence. Some things have worked, while others have not (this does not mean that these things will not work for another person). I will list everything I have tried below, along with their purpose:

- Tights puller upper – I used this tool to help myself pull up my tights (Fig. 20.1).

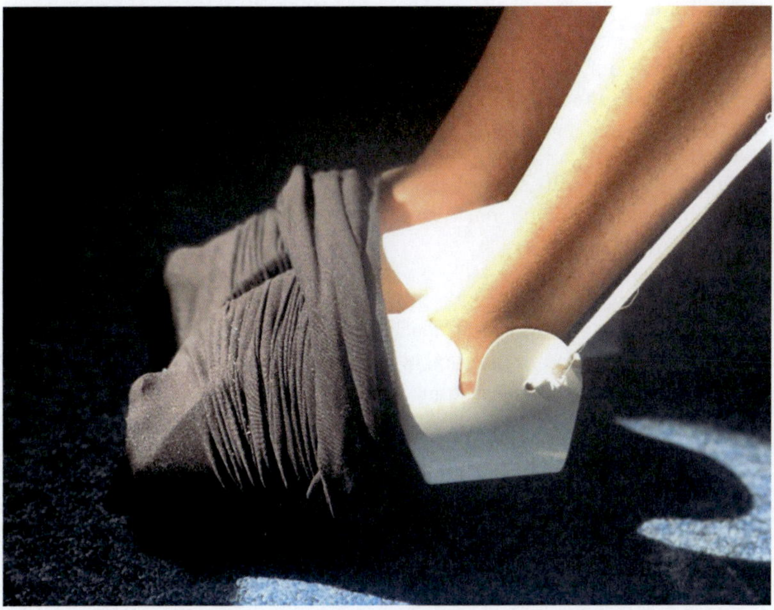

Fig. 20.1. Tights puller upper. © Bianca Wiersema. Reproduced with permission from the author.

While using the tights puller, I encountered the following problems:

- It was very difficult to put both feet in the aid— as I put one foot in, the other foot came out, resulting in even more spasticity in the feet.
- If I managed to put both feet in the aid, the tool would occasionally come out of the tights and I would have to take it from the beginning. As a result, the body's spasticity increased.
- If the tights are too tight or too wide, the aid becomes unstable and they fall out from the aid.
- AIf I managed to put my feet in and not let the aid run out of the tights, the force that the aid required me to have was greater than I could handle (because I was generally with my legs outstretched and the tights could not slide on the leg), which resulted in greater spasticity in the hands and trapezius muscle; also, my hands became tired, which resulted in the release of one of the parts of the support (to effectively pull the aid, you should pull it with both hands at the same time), which resulted in the execution of the movements from the start.

When pulling your tights with the aid, you must lean forward enough to be able to pull the support, which can cause an increase in back spasticity and lower back pain.

Grabbing stick (Fig. 20.2.) – I used this tool to put on my socks as well as to grab things. They come in a variety of sizes. I encountered the following difficulties when using it:

- When I pulled on one side of the sock, the other side slipped.
- If the sock was too tight, I was not able to fit all of my toes into it, and if I tried to put the sock on one toe at a time, the sock slipped off the toes on which it was placed.
- When I managed to put the sock on, it did not sit comfortably on the toes and heels.
- When attempting to put on the sock, it was a great effort for my hands, which, if excessive, can result in increased spasticity in the hands.

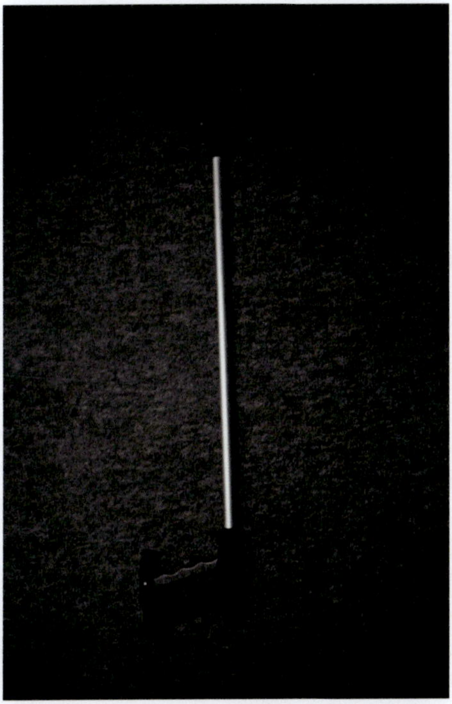

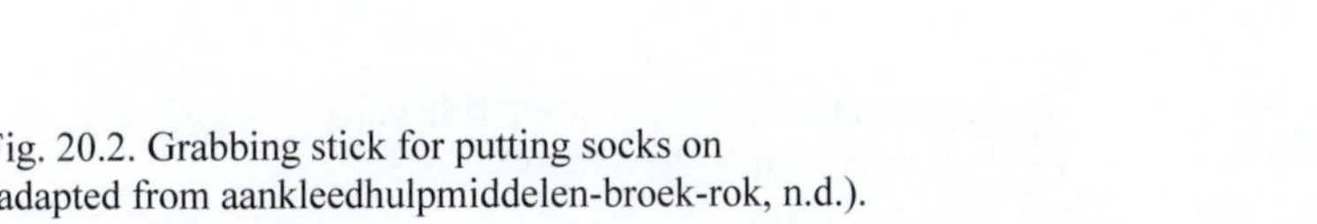

Fig. 20.2. Grabbing stick for putting socks on
(adapted from aankleedhulpmiddelen-broek-rok, n.d.).

➢ Pants dressing aid (Fig. 20.3.) – I attempted to put on trousers using the device below, but it was inefficient. Even if I was able to put my legs in the trousers, in order to be able to pull them up, I had to stand up, keep myself balanced with one hand on something fixed, and with the other hand to pull the elastic that held the trousers, which unbalanced me even more. When I pulled on one side of the trousers, the other side of the trousers fell down, just like with the socks.

- I pull my trousers up by pulling the trousers' loop on one side with one hand while keeping myself balanced with the other hand hand on something fixed and then pull the loop on the other side until I manage to pull them all the way up.

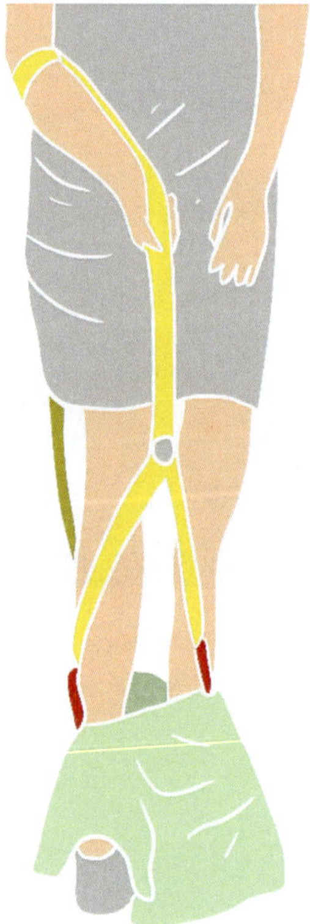

Fig. 20.3. This image depicts a Clip-n-Pull device to help pull the trousers up (adapted from Clip-n-Pull: Pants Assist Dressing Aid, n.d.).

When I was younger because of the spasticity in my jaw, which prevents this movement, I was unable to suck on a baby bottle. (A pacifier is also not used for this purpose). For me, spoon-feeding was effective in this situation.

Because a person cannot defend himself, he may be afraid of any movement, including animals and birds and it may take more time to adjust to such things.

As I mentioned in previous chapters, I support a person's independence in various ways, but a balance between independence and spasticity must be found. If you try to achieve something and see that after several attempts, the person cannot do it, try to focus on what the person can do and make that fruitful. At the same time, learn to accept both the person who achieves these things and the individual who takes care of him and helps him that some things cannot be done for various reasons. This, although difficult to accept, will save you a lot of nervous breakdowns, frustrations, and time. On the other hand, you will learn to appreciate the small things that can be accomplished, and that successes do not have to be grandiose to be valuable. Time, persistence, and many failures have taught me that it is not how many times you fail that matters, but what you learn from each failure in order to get back up and try again. I am convinced that learning to live with a disability marks the end of limitations and the beginning of versatility and that there is a lesson waiting to be learned in every experience we have.

CHAPTER 21

HOW TO DEAL WITH CONSTIPATION

In this chapter I will discuss various methods that helped me deal with constipation (the laxatives I used are discussed in Chapter 16). The following are some of them:

- Cereals with oats and fruit served with milk or yogurt.
- Buckwheat and rye with milk or yogurt.
- Plums with or without yogurt.

I have buckwheat and rye with yogurt every morning, and plums during the day to favor digestion.

In general, I eat dried plums, but when they are in season (summer-autumn), I also eat them fresh.

You can try to combine what you like and see what helps you best with your digestion.

It is important to have diverse and balanced food so that you can have balanced levels of nutrients in your body.

For me, the effect of evacuation has diminished after 3 weeks of eating, let's say, plums because my body has gotten used to it, so I try to switch between different approaches.

- Drink senna tea in small quantities because it can cause severe diarrhea.

Since I have been able to eat on my own, I have used cutlery; I never ate with my hands or with adjusted cutlery. It is important for a child to eat with a normal spoon because it will be easier for him to also eat in a restaurant because it gets him accustomed to the world outside the house. I cannot eat raw carrots, raw potatoes, fruits with harder skin, hard corners of bread, food with a hard crust, almonds, or hard meat because chewing them causes contractions in my jaw, but I can eat soft foods like any vegetable and cooked meat, as well as soft fruits (oranges, grapes, bananas). As apples are more difficult to bite, I prefer to eat them sliced. I also prefer to eat liver mashed or combined with puree rather than whole because it is easier to chew.

i. Gaining and losing weight

I struggled with my weight a lot, especially as a student, and it had a big impact on my body. Weight gain or loss can affect the body's spasticity. The issues I encountered and their impact on my overall functioning are described in detail below. Gaining too much weight in comparison to one's height may have the following consequences:

- Pain in the lower back (this pain can lead to an increase in spasticity in that area).
- Problems with maintaining balance - keeping your balance becomes more difficult as well as repositioning your body in an upright position.
- Getting out of bed takes more time and is done with greater effort, which leads to an increase in spasticity in the hands, as well as in the rest of the body.
- When compared to when you were thinner, breathing is more difficult, especially when making an effort, and you feel as if you are running out of air. Weight gain promotes breathing difficulties due to the extra effort required, BUT it does not cause an increase in spasticity in the chest on its own. Breathing difficulties can intensify by increased spasticity in the chest, but the problem can be solved with physiotherapy and weight loss.
- When you do exercises, you get tired faster and you require more breaks to recover.
- You notice that your legs are no longer supporting you while walking.

In general, the body makes much more effort to perform the same tasks as before, which leads to an increase in body spasticity and thus pain. In addition to physical difficulties, you may also face:

- Fatigue
- Sweating
- Sleeping problems
- Irascibility / irritability
- Unhappiness, etc.

Additionally, weight loss can lead to a loss of muscle mass and thus strength, which can lead to:

- Difficulties in maintaining balance.
- Muscle weakness that results in the inability of the body to perform a movement that involves the use of muscles that have lost strength.

The following are some of the advantages of having a stable and well-proportioned weight in relation to one's height:

- Maintaining body balance for a longer period of time.
- Breathing issues are less frequent.
- It is a lot easier to get out of bed.
- When you make an effort you do not get tired so fast.
- Physiotherapy sessions leave you feeling energized rather than exhausted.
- You have the energy to carry out more activities (you do not become so tired after performing an activity).

From the point of view of someone who has tried numerous diets to lose weight, the most successful diet was to minimize the amount of food consumed rather than to completely eliminate pasta, chocolate or bread. I eat a wide variety of foods, but in smaller portions. Furthermore, alcohol intake was only rarely, combined with 30-40 minutes of daily physical training (physiotherapy sessions are a bonus in addition to daily physical activity), which increases the body's mobility. Establishing daily routine exercises is the secret to maintaining good mobility. If you do not develop a physical routine, your body will become more spastic by the day.

It is best to avoid physical activity when you are tired because both your ability to focus and the quality of your workouts will suffer. Inadequate exercise can cause discomfort, which can lead to an increase in spasticity in the body.

ii. Caffeine

Moderate coffee consumption has advantages, but excessive consumption or combining it with other caffeinated beverages can have the following consequences:

- Your heart rate increases and you might begin to shake.

- You may begin to sweat and feel cold as a result. The cold will cause an increase in spasticity and, as a result, an increase in pain.
- Caffeine consumption may cause agitation, which can lead to more frequent contractions in the body, resulting in increased spasticity and pain (effects that can be felt a few hours after drinking coffee).

These effects are the ones I have experienced, but there are others and each person is unique in the manifestations they can experience.

According to mine, try not to drink coffee at least 3 hours before your physiotherapy session, so that your body has time to eliminate the caffeine (after drinking coffee, try to drink water to avoid dehydration). If you drink coffee shortly before your physiotherapy session, you will experience increased spasticity and find it more difficult to coordinate your movements during the physiotherapy session (and you will relax even harder).

CHAPTER 22

THE REVIVAL OF INDIVIDUALITY, DISABILITY AND SEX

I chose to study the minor "Gender and Sexuality in Society and Culture" as part of my university curriculum. We discussed some controversial topics, such as what gender/sexuality is and what defines it, or how society views gender and sexuality that does not conform to the heterosexual norm that we are expected to follow. But the theme that has impressed me the most is how people with a disability have the right to express their sexuality and are allowed to desire and be desired by others. And then a work of Eli Clare's entitled "Gawking, Gaping, Staring" found its way into my hands. He emphasizes what we often overlook: people that have a disability are still people who want to love and be loved. In someone else's eyes, what we consider to be flaws can be something beautiful and cherished if you learn to discover the person and look beyond the disability, an idea Clare presents as follows: "we are looking for...lovers to reach beneath our clothes, beneath the words that attempt to name us, beneath our shame and armor, their eyes and hands helping return us to grace, beauty, and passion."(Clare, 2003, 258).

Even though it is a taboo subject, sex and sexuality represent needs that everyone has and should express in his own, unique way. I want to dispel the myth that people that have a disability are asexual or do not have sexual desires; they simply express their sexuality and sexual desires in a different way than we are used to. If you want to know a person's sexual needs and desires (whether he has a disability or not), ask that person, even if the question appears inappropriate to you, it is the only way to be honest, and take into account the person's point of view. On November 27th 2021, Life in Progress website by Adriana Galatar describes best what I want to say: "People in wheelchairs have a lot to offer and, at the end of the day, sex is done with the person, not with his chair."

You can use the wheelchair to foster creativity or spice up your sexual experience, as long as you put the brakes on to avoid slipping away or falling backward.

Some people break the bed, others break the wheelchair.

Open communication, no matter how difficult it is, is the key to a healthy relationship, whether or not sex is involved.

The presence of a sexual relationship between two people does not always imply the presence of a couple relationship. In other words, you can be sexually intimate with someone without having a relationship with him or her, and this is neither good nor bad; it is simply different.

Another issue I would like to bring up is that some people want to have sex with a person who has a disability just to brag in the eyes of others. If you find yourself in this situation, talk to appropriate persons, try not to be alone with that individual for too long, and inform another appropriate person about the individual you are meeting.

According to Amy Connors, sexual orientation, desires, preferences, and kinks still differ from person to person regardless of physical limitations and sexuality. Additionally, people who have a disability, experience sexual frustration on the same level like everyone else. Many people dislike the idea of thinking of people who have a disability as sexual because it reminds them of their physical vulnerabilities and they may be afraid of taking advantage of the person who has a disability. It reminds them of their flaws because the majority of physical limitations are associated with the aging process.

A lot of people want to think they are invincible especially when they are younger but people who have a disability are forced to acknowledge the reality much quicker (Amy Connors, Discord message to Bianca Wiersema, July 27-28, 2022).

While many people consider sexuality to be a taboo topic, this should not preclude you from enjoying it and exploring it in different ways. The challenge we face nowadays, whether we are a woman, a man, disabled, or have any other sexual identity that does not fit the norm, is the ability to be ourselves, embrace our weaknesses and strengths, and speak up. If we want to change people's perceptions of gender, sex, disability, and sexual identity, we must first tear down boundaries and rebuild a boundless space of development. This, in my opinion, is best expressed by Loree Erickson's words: "The problem is not with the disabled person, the problem is the environment. Disability is diversity, not a deficit." (Ansari, 2013).

CHAPTER 23

FINDING A CURE

SARDARU DRAGOȘ

Cerebral palsy is a term that means "brain paralysis." It is a movement and body position disability. It results from brain damage that occurred prior to the baby's birth, during birth, or as a baby. Only parts of the brain, primarily those that control movement, are affected. Once damaged, brain areas do not recover or worsen. However, depending on how we treat the child and how damaged his or her brain is, the child's movements, body positions, and related problems can be improved or worsened. The earlier we start, the better improvements we can make (Werner, 1987, chap. 9).

The main objective of physical therapy is to prevent disease rather than cure it. The primary goal should be to reduce spasticity while improving quality of life and general functioning.

Some physical therapists massage or rub the affected area in an attempt to relax tense muscles. Frequent massages relieve muscle spasms, cramps, or tight muscles. However, in cases of spasticity, a massage typically tightens the muscles. MASSAGE OF SPASTIC MUSCLES IS NOT ADVISABLE IN GENERAL. (Werner, 1987, chap. 9).

The first rule in therapy is to help as much as necessary, while encouraging the person to do as much as possible by himself (Werner, 1987, chap. 35).

The techniques described below had been used in the case of spastic tetraparesis. Keep in mind that these are only guidelines and that the physiotherapy and rehabilitation programme must be customized according to the patient's medical condition and needs.

The techniques generally applied are used after the **P**roprioceptive **N**euromuscular **F**acilitation (PNF) Kabat concept for neuro-reeducation.

For the upper limbs:

Rhythmical initiation and rhythmical rotation for the relaxation of the shoulder, elbow and the wrist of the hand. Rhythmical initiation is done the first time passively and after that the patient is beginning to help finish with the resistance for the patterns that are needed to be empowered.

Rhythmical initiation on the patterns of: Flex+Abd+ER and Ext+Abd+IR. On these models I also stretch the muscle chains that are spastic. I target for stretching and relaxation of these muscles: Flexors of the hand, flexors of the elbow and pronators muscles, pectoralis major and minor muscles, coracobrachialis muscle, latissimus dorsi, trapezius, levator scapulae muscle.

PNF – Hold-Relax + stretching the flexor and pronator muscles of the hand, elbow flexors, and internal rotation of the shoulder.

Easy rhythmic mobilizations for the fist, elbow, and shoulder joints (first passive, then active-passive, then active-assisted).

PNF – Hold-Relax + stretching for trapezius, scalenes and sternocleidomastoid.

PNF – Shoulder diagonal as follows:

Diagonal 1 in the flexion pattern: shoulder flexion, adduction, and external rotation.

Diagonal 1 in the extension pattern: extension, abduction, and internal rotation.

Diagonal 2 in the flexion pattern: flexion, abduction, and external rotation.

Diagonal 2 in the extension pattern: extension, adduction, and internal rotation.

The movements are performed first passive, then active-assisted, active with resistance, and Hold-Relax.

Massage of the face, effleurage, friction, and stretching (easy, harder maneuvers alternated with easier ones), in case of an increase in spasticity at the face.

Combination of isotonics also on the same patterns working the normal muscles.

Hold-Relax (reciprocal inhibition) and other techniques that are derived from it (Muscle energy techniques, Post isometric relaxation – which are basically the same things but used in the branch of osteopathy) are used for the diminution of the spasticity. And also, positional reflexes of the head, neck, and trunk to inhibit the pathological neural flow.

Asymmetrical model pattern to counteract the patient's reflex of moving both upper limbs at the same time.

Functional workout on the same patterns in which the patient is asked to locate and retrieve different objects in variable positions together with the main patterns.

Mobilization of the scapulae complex and the cervical spine. Here I have also used Hold-Relax, combined with stretching = PNF stretching.

Massage with movement technique for spastic muscles.

Transverse frictional massage (Cyriax) and sometimes Shiatsu on trigger points.

Massage of the back, rubbing, friction, pressure, and vibrations.

For the lower limbs:

Rhythmical initiation and rhythmical rotation for the relaxation of the coxofemural muscles.

PNF stretching combined with reciprocal inhibition (Hold-Relax) on: psoas-iliac muscles ++, hamstring muscles group, gastrocnemius, and soleus muscles.

Repeated stretch technique with progressive resistance for foot dorsiflexion.

Functional workout on different patterns.

PNF – Hold-Relax + stretching on the dorsiflexion muscles of the foot, plantar flexion of the foot, knee extension, thigh flexion on the hip, thigh extension, and thigh internal rotation.

Easy rhythmic mobilizations for the ankle, knee and hip joints.

PNF – Hip diagonal as shown below:

Diagonal 1 for the hip in the flexion pattern: flexion, adduction, and external rotation.

Diagonal 1 in the extension pattern: extension, abduction, and internal rotation.

Diagonal 2 in the flexion pattern: flexion, abduction, and internal rotation.

Diagonal 2 in the extension pattern: extension, adduction, and external rotation.

The movements are performed in the following order: passive, active-assisted, active with resistance, and Hold-Relax.

Stretching for the lumbar muscles

One hand opposes the resistance on the dorsal part of the paw of one leg, the other hand opposes the resistance on the plantar side of the other leg - the sockets are changed at the same time at the end of the race - after a certain number of repetitions, isometry will be done.

For the trunk:

Stretch techniques on: erector spinae muscles, quadratus lumborum muscles, trapezius muscles….sometimes intercostalis muscles when the patient is really tensed.

Massage with movement technique for the lower part of the erector spinae muscles.

Working on the equilibrium:

Assisted walking, in front of the patient, the patient must be supported and guided. He will take the next step only when he straightens his pelvis. The patient has to look ahead while walking.

While standing in front of the patient, supported and guided, he will lift and hold each leg up for as long as possible, and he will control his pelvis to be in a neutral position.

While standing in front of the patient, supported and guided, slightly unbalance the patient while supporting him and he will have to rebalance himself.

Destabilization of different girdles in a quadruped position, in sitting position (on a Swiss ball) and standing position.

Walking freely in different patterns and with an elastic suit that challenges to activate the proprioceptors of the patient.

The patient's cooperation in re-education is critical to achieving results in functional re-education; all treatment will be determined by the person's intelligence quotient (Gotia and Ardelean, 1993, 157).

CHAPTER 24

FINAL WORDS

People with this type of diagnosis, but not only, struggle from a young age to obtain basic life necessities such as the ability to eat, breathe, grab different things to satisfy a need, go to the toilet, and so on. It takes time and effort to achieve mobility and independence in life, and thus a higher quality of life. Failures and regression are unavoidable, but they are necessary for learning how to move forward and focus on what the person can develop and use. Because these people fall more frequently, they learn to get back up and go further; however, upon closer examination, this becomes an asset, as they have learned to deal with whatever they have at hand in any situation and to use their creativity and inventiveness when challenged. People who do not have medical problems that prevent them from meeting their basic needs and thus have not learned to fall and then learn how to get back up; when these people fall, figuratively or literally, they either do not know how to become stronger or give up without even attempting, turning them into people defeated by their own ideals and trapped in their own limitations.

There is no one who can decide what is normal and what is not. So many times have I heard the phrase, "they, because they are normal, can...and you, because you are disabled, cannot do what they do." However, if you take a closer look around, you will notice that the people you call healthy can have worse problems than the person that the world says is different. But the person who you say is different from the rest usually possesses special and unique abilities that by far outweigh the expectations of others. This is the same special person who, when others struggle with difficulties – and they run, give up, freeze, and come up with a million reasons why it would not work or why they will not make it – moves forward and faces everything that comes his way, reacts and does not freeze, looks for solutions, rather than obstacles, and gets up every time he falls. This person finds out and understands early in life that you can learn to dance in the rain and that the sun always rises after each storm. This person knows that asking for help when you need it makes you stronger because he has faced more challenges than others. He has become tougher and more resilient and will not give up so easily on what life throws at him.

Before judging anybody, keep in mind that all you really know about them is their name, not their story. If you really want to know somebody, be brave and ask them. Life is not measured in years, but in simple moments that become infinite memories. Being unique does not have to be a negative thing. It can imply that you have the courage and insanity to be yourself and overcome your boundaries when everyone else is busy copying with the world around them and content to live within their own boundaries. That because you exist, small miracles happen.

I think David Werner expressed very well my idea, which he presents as following: "The challenge, whenever possible, should be to build on the unique strengths, experience, and qualities of the disabled person: help her to find a role in society that she can do better than most non-disabled persons. Disability does make a person different in certain ways, for better and for worse. Rather than pretending that the difference does not exist, it is wiser to accept the differences and look for ways that being disabled helps to deepen or strengthen the person. Help the person to have not just an ordinary role in society, but one that is in some ways outstanding." (Werner, 1987, chap. 54).

Wherever I went in Romania (hospitals, schools, hotels), the lack of accessibility was always an impediment but also a challenge, necessitating the discovery of innovative ways to reach the destination.

The assistive aids should be used only when needed to increase independence. Too much reliance on them can make the person dependent on them, making him less independent and therefore less self-supported.

I will end with a quote that belongs to Tedy Necula, namely: "People need inspiration, aiming to be inspired by themselves." (Necula, T., 2018).

CHAPTER 25

THANKS

The names of some of the professionals who assisted me along the way are provided below in the hope that they will assist others as well.

- Prof. Dr. Cristian Dinu, Popescu – Primary Neurologist Doctor- passed away in 2017
- Prof. Dr. Dorin, Chisăliță- Primary Ophthalmologist – for strabismus
- Dr. Ioan, Petcu – Primary Orthopedic Doctor
- Dr. Maria, Colonescu- Primary Pediatric Doctor
- Prof. Dr. Maria, Stamatin – Primary Neonatalogist Doctor
- Prof. Dr. Sebastian, Cozma – Primary ENT Doctor
- Joshua, Dickerson – for choosing the right wheelchair https://www.southwestmedical.com/
- Van Mossel, Hoortolstellen- Leiderdorp - for hearing aids https://www.vanmosselhoortoestellen.nl/

APPENDICES

Appendix A- Medical history and surgeries

- Medical history

The patient came from a pregnancy with problems (the cervix opened at 4 months, with externalization of the membranes), born prematurely at 26 weeks, with a birth weight of 1000 g. She had a delay in psycho-motor development (holding her head at 3 years, sitting at 5 years and started walking at 11 years old with unilateral support). She underwent 3 surgeries in the past for lengthening tendons (adductors at 4 years, Achille's at 7 years, semimembranosus at 11 years), and had several injections of botulinum toxin in 2011 (interrupted due to intense dry headaches).

Neurological exam: upper arm in flexion and pronation: lower arm in external rotation; bilateral amblyopia; strabismus; bilateral hypoacusis; standing and walking impossible; tetraparetic motor deficit; elastic hypertonia in upper limbs and lower limbs; r.o.t. members and patellae vii bilaterally; diminished Achilles; Babinski (+) bilaterally; Rossolimo (+) bilaterally; cervical and back pain on palpation; bilateral leg hypotrophy.

- Tenotomy of bilateral Achilles lengthening and immobilization in a bilateral cruro-podal cast device

SUMMARY OF THE MEDICAL CHART

(Epicrisis, recommendations)

The 6-year-old patient known with IMOC (spastic tetraparesis), predominantly on the lower limbs, equine spastic foot, bilateral irreducible.

Percutaneous tenotomy of bilateral Achilles lengthening and immobilization in a bilateral cruro-podal gypsum apparatus was performed.

- Tenotomy of the tibial-hamstring muscle of the bilateral knee.

SUMMARY OF THE MEDICAL CHART

(Epicrisis, recommendations)

The 9-year-old patient known with IMOC (spastic tetraparesis) for which she suffered from surgeries at the level of the hip and bilateral foot in early childhood refers to our clinic for periodical examination.

The clinical examination sets out the above-mentioned diagnoses. We performed a tenotomy of the tibial-hamstring muscle of the bilateral knee with the correction of the bilateral flexion and immobilization in gypsum cruro-hamstring apparatus on both sides was also required, which the patient tolerated well.

Favorable post-surgery evolution.

Recommendations

- Maintains the gypsum immobilization for 3 weeks.
- Continues the cruro-hamstring immobilization (fixed orthosis) in a continuous regime and in a discontinuous regime for 6 months afterwards.
- Returns for examination after 3 weeks post-surgery.

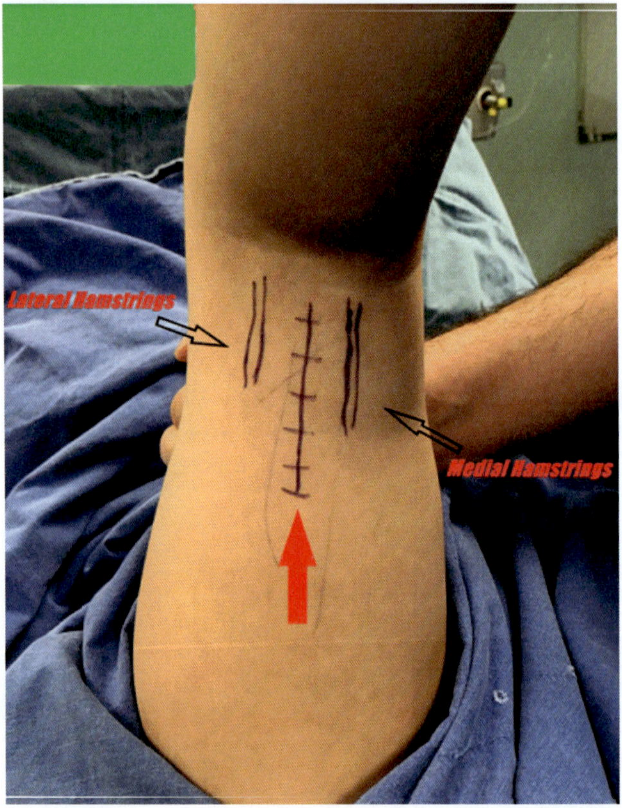

Appendix A-Fig.1. The midline incision for the open hamstring lengthening (red arrow) and traces of medial and lateral hamstring muscle groups (Clinical Comparison of Percutaneous and Open Hamstring Lengthening in Children with Spastic Cerebral Palsy, Medeniyet Medical Journal, 2019, 184). © Medeniyet Medical Journal. Reproduced with permission from the publisher.

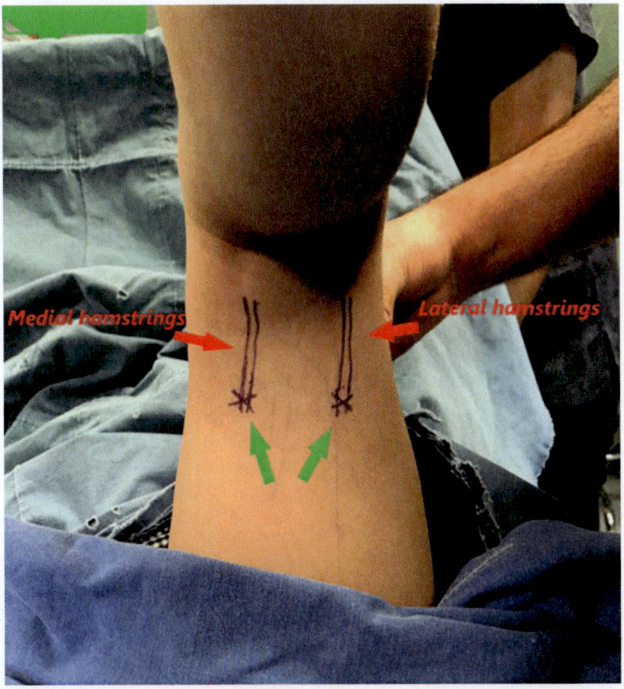

Appendix A-Fig.2. The traces of medial and lateral hamstring muscle groups and the entry points of surgical blades for percutaneous hamstring lengthening (green arrows) (left lower extremity; hip is flexed 90° and the knee joint is in maximum extension). (Clinical Comparison of Percutaneous and Open Hamstring Lengthening in Children with Spastic Cerebral Palsy, Medeniyet Medical Journal, 2019, 184). © Medeniyet Medical Journal. Reproduced with permission from the publisher.

➢ Gastrocnemius elongation tenotomy

SUMMARY OF THE MEDICAL CHART

(Discharge summary, recommendations)

Admitted according to the schedule with the above mentioned diagnoses, 10 June 2013.

The patient was subject to surgery under rachianesthesia. Bilateral gastrocnemius elongation tenotomy (Strayer technique) was performed and immobilization in a cruro-podal circular gypsum apparatus with the knee in extension and the leg in a position of dorsal correction was also required. The patient tolerated the immobilization well.

Plain post-surgery evolution, without complications.

Recommendations

- Maintains the bilateral cruro-podal immobilization for 3 weeks;
- Examination with a referral for suppressing the wires and changing the bilateral gypsum apparatus;
- TVP prophylaxis with Fraxiparine 0.4 ml injection s.c. per day, for 6 weeks (this was recommended by the orthopedic doctor, who performed the surgery and the doses are personalized to the person).

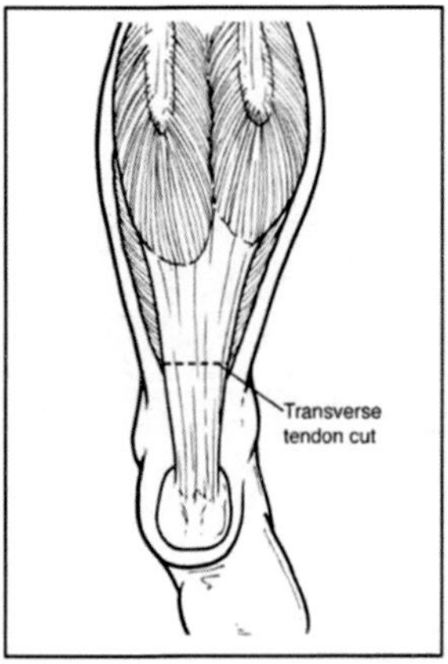

Appendix A-Fig.3.Diagram showing the level of transaction for a strayer procedure (TECHNIQUES OF GASTROCNEMIUS RECESSION, Update 2004, The Podiatry Institute, 172). © The Podiatry Institute. Reproduced with permission from the publisher.

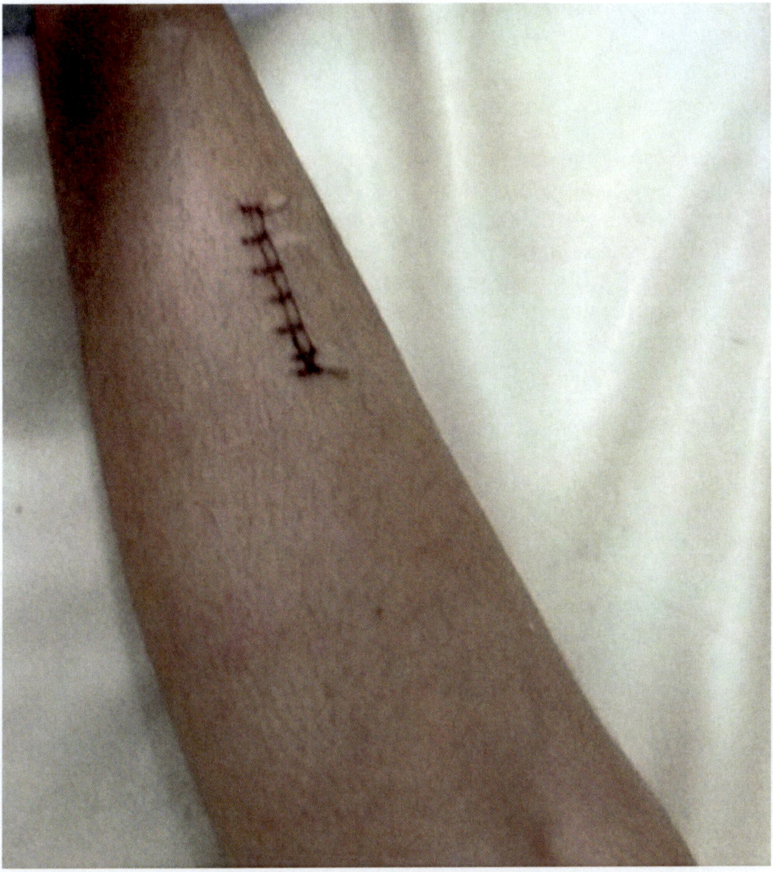

Appendix A-Fig.4-This image shows the incision of the Achille's tendon, post-surgery. © Bianca Wiersema. Reproduced with permission from the author.

Appendix B- Botulinum toxin and side effects.

In 2011, the patient came with the diagnosis: Chronic infantile encephalopathy; Spastic tetraparesis.

Ex neurological: upper limbs in flexion and pronation; lower limbs in flexion and external rotation; hearing loss; low visual acuity in both eyes; walking possible with unilateral support, difficult for short distances, spastic and bilateral scissoring; upper and lower limbs motor deficit; left upper limb> right upper limb; elastic hypertonia in upper limbs and lower limbs with limitation of flexion-extension and pronation – supination movements; dysmetria with PIN hypermetria on the left; ROT upper limbs vii bilaterally; ROT vii patellar clonoid achillenes.

1000 U of Dysport were injected in the right and left brachial upper limbs, right and left supinator, right and left semimembranous lower limbs, gastrocnemius 2 right and 2 left points.

The likelihood of having an adverse reaction is described by the following groups:

Very common - occur in more than 1 in 10 patients treated
Common - less than 1 in 10 patients treated
Less common - less than 1 in 100 patients treated
Rare - less than 1 in 1000 patients treated

Treatment of any disease (all patients)

Side effects that have occurred include:

Common: bruising or pain around the injection site or a burning sensation at the time of injection, general weakness, tiredness, flu-like symptoms.

Less common: itching.

Rare: rash and muscle weakness.

Other adverse reactions related to the diffusion of Dysport away from the site of administration have also been reported (worsening of muscle weakness, difficulty swallowing or breathing, which, in very rare cases were fatal).

During the course of treatment for upper limb spasticity

Treatment-related adverse reactions are typically mild to moderate in severity.

These are transient reactions that usually occur within the first few weeks of injection.

- Localized and, in rare cases, generalized muscle weakness is the most common side effect. Muscle weakness is caused by the expected pharmacological action of botulinum toxin after injection.
- Flu-like symptoms, fatigue and drowsiness, and pain at the injection site have also been reported.
- Other side effects observed in clinical trials include: gait disturbances, injection site bruising, bleeding, muscle and bone pain, pain in hands and fingers, muscle spasms, and difficulty swallowing.

Treatment for arm muscle spasms

Among the adverse reactions that have occurred are:

- Muscle weakness and musculoskeletal pain are the most common symptoms.
- Pain in the extremities is less common.

Adults with lower limb spasticity

- Muscle weakness in the legs, muscle pain, difficulty swallowing, weakness, fatigue, flu-like illness, and injection site reactions are all common (pain, bruising, rash, itching) symptoms (Anm.ro., n.d.).

Bibliography

Amazon.de. n.d. "Heated Trousers Electric Heating Trousers with 3 Adjustable Temperature USB Charging, Heated Thermal Trousers for Men Women Outdoor Hiking Hunting Motorcycle Camping (Batteries Not Included), Black Men, XL Slim Kurz : Amazon.de: Fashion", black men, XL Slim Kurz." Amazon.de. Accessed May 14, 2023. https://www.amazon.de/-/en/Trousers-Adjustable-Temperature-Motorcycle-Batteries/dp/B0987VNSB4/ref=sr_1_5?adgrpid=108692620481&dchild=1&gclid=CjwKCAjwhaaKBhBcEiwA8acsHLgAdWBECBq7tYRuEHe2xXA9j7U-vZidbZw4t5Iq8HsNpKVcJLNMZxoCFSQQAvD_BwE&hvadid=451300454546&hvdev=c&hvlocphy=1011828&hvnetw=g&hvqmt=e&hvrand=3303064015317787144&hvtargid=kwd-506155551272&hydadcr=5178_1985503&keywords=beheizbare%2Bhose&qid=1632225644&sr=8-5.

Amazon.com. n.d. "Vive Forearm Crutches (Pair) - Lightweight Arm Cuff Crutch - Adjustable, Ergonomic, Heavy Duty for Standard and Tall Adults - Comfortable on Wrist - Molded, Non Skid Replaceable Rubber Tips : Health & Household." Amazon.com. Accesed May 24, 2023. https://www.amazon.com/Forearm-Crutches-Vive-Pair-Lightweight/dp/B06X3XQ6QK

Ansari, Aeman. 2013. "Disability Is a Diversity, Not a Deficit." The Eyeopener. Accessed May 17, 2023. https://theeyeopener.com/2013/04/disability-is-a-diversity-not-a-deficit/#comments.

Apgar, Virginia, Duncan A Holaday, Stanley James, Irvin, M. Weisbrot. 1958. "Evaluation of the Newborn Infant-Second Report." *Journal of the American Medical Association* 168, No. 15:1-4. https://doi.org/10.1001/jama.1958.03000150027007.

Archie, Hinchcliffe. 2007. "Assessing a Child with Cerebral Palsy: II. Analysis of Observations." In Children with Cerebral Palsy: A Manual for Therapists, Parents and Community Workers, 50–70. https://doi.org/10.4135/9788132108528.n3

Anm.ro. n.d. "Autorizaţie de Punere Pe Piaţă nr. 10661/2018/01 anexa 1 ... – ANMDMR." Accessed May 15, 2023. https://www.anm.ro/_/_PRO/PRO_10661_15.03.18.pdf

"Baston CU 3 Picioare." Toda International SRL. Accessed May 11, 2023. https://echipamenteortopedice.ro/baston-cu-3-sau-4-picioare/20-baston-cu-3-picioare.html?gclid=CjwKCAjwuIWHBhBDEiwACXQYsf94rR2WFhcLpF62yHloZNA4TI-TSZ4IDWv-VOyZCDmPMFDr-Y8TQxoC13MQAvD_BwE

"Baston Din Lemn Cu Maner Clasic." Catena Pas cu Pas. Accessed May 8, 2023. https://www.catenapascupas.ro/baston-din-lemn-cu-maner-clasic

Beers, M. H. 2004. *The Merck manual of medical information*: Second home edition. Simon and Schuster.

Bio Terra Med. 2016. "Deviațiile de Ax Ale Genunchilor (Ii) Bio Terra Med." Bio Terra Med. Accessed May 17.https://bioterramed.ro/deviatiile-de-ax-ale-genunchilor-ii/.

"Cadru de Mers Cu Rotile." Toda International SRL. Accessed May 11, 2023. https://echipamenteortopedice.ro/cadru-de-mers/54-cadru-de-mers-cu-rotile.html.

Chandrasekhar, Annapoorna, Noor Azuan Abu Osman, Lai Kuan Tham, Kheng Seang Lim, and Wan Abu Wan Abas. 2013."Influence of Age on Patellar Tendon Reflex Response." *PLoS ONE* 8, No. 11. e80799. https://doi.org/10.1371/journal.pone.0080799.

Chung, Sun G., Elton M. van Rey, Zhiqiang Bai, Mark W. Rogers, Elliot J. Roth, and Li-Qun Zhang. 2005. "Aging-Related Neuromuscular Changes Characterized by Tendon Reflex System Properties." *Archives of Physical Medicine and Rehabilitation* 86, No. 2: 318–27. https://doi.org/10.1016/j.apmr.2004.04.048.

Clare, Eli. 2003."Gawking, Gaping, Staring." *GLQ: A Journal of Lesbian and Gay Studies* 9, No. 1–2: 257–61. https://doi.org/10.1215/10642684-9-1-2-257.

Cocco, Antoniangela, and Alberto Albanese. 2018."Recent Developments in Clinical Trials of Botulinum Neurotoxins." *Toxicon* 147: 77–83. https://doi.org/10.1016/j.toxicon.2017.08.014.

Cohen, P, and J G Kohn. 1979."Follow-up Study of Patients with Cerebral Palsy." *The Western Journal of Medicine* 130, No. 1: 6–11.

Cosgrove, A. P., I. S. Corry, and H. K. Graham. 2008. "Botulinum Toxin in the Management of the Lower Limb in Cerebral Palsy". 2008. *Developmental Medicine & Child Neurology* 36, No. 5: 386–96. https://doi.org/10.1111/j.1469-8749.1994.tb11864.x.

Cîrstoveanu, Catalin. 2020." Încercăm Să Ne Uităm Care Este Primul Care Moare Pe Listă Şi PE Acela Îl Luăm" / „Minunile Apar Acolo Unde Este Foarte Multă Muncă"."Interview by Mara Raducan. Mediafax, October 21, 2020. https://www.mediafax.ro/stirile-zilei/ochii-mine-doctorul-catalin-cirstoveanu-dragostea-copii-batalia-pat-terapie-intensiva-incercam-ne-uitam-primul-moare-lista-acela-il-luam-minunile-apar-acolo-unde-foarte-multa-munca-19686685.

Cruickshank, W.M.1976. (Ed.), Cerebral palsy:A developmental disability. Syracuse, N.Y.: Syracuse University Press.

Dafkin, Chloe, Andrew Green, Samantha Kerr, Demetri Veliotes, and Warrick Mckinon. 2012. "The Accuracy of Subjective Clinical Assessments of the Patellar Reflex." *Muscle & Nerve* 47, No. 1: 81–88. https://doi.org/10.1002/mus.23487.

Davis, Bill. 2019. "A Comprehensive Comparison Guide: Paralysis vs. Paresis." Thriving With Paralysis. Accessed May 17, 2023. https://www.thrivingwithparalysis.com/comparison-paralysis-vs-paresis/.

Denhoff, Eric.1976. Medical aspects. In W. M. Cruickshank (Ed.), *Cerebral palsy: A developmental disability*. Syracuse, N.Y.: Syracuse University Press.

Diaconu, Georgeta. 2008." Paraliziile cerebrale". In *PEDIATRIE- patologie digestivă, nutriţională şi neurologică la copil*, edited by Moraru, D., Burlea, M., Moraru, E., Cîrdei, E., & Diaconu, Georgeta, 247-257. Iași, RO: Fundația Academică AXIS.

Dinf.ne.jp. n.d. "Disabled Village Children." Disabled Village Children - CONTENTS. Accessed May 15, 2023. https://www.dinf.ne.jp/doc/english/global/david/dwe002/dwe00201.html.

Duncan, Pamela W., and Mary Beth Badke. 1987. *Stroke rehabilitation: The recovery of motor control.* Chicago: Year Book Medical Publishers.

Fasen, Madeline, Brittany Saldivar, Suhane Elamsenthil, Jordan Thompson, Lina Fouad, Linda Edwards, and Rafik Jacob.2020. "Gynecological Care and Contraception Considerations in Women with Cerebral Palsy." *Southern Medical Journal* 113, No. 11: 549–52. https://doi.org/10.14423/smj.0000000000001170.

Fontana, L. 2011. "Thermal Performance of Radiant Heating Floors in Furnished Enclosed Spaces." *Applied Thermal Engineering* 31, No. 10: 1547–55. https://doi.org/10.1016/j.applthermaleng.2010.12.014.

Fortuna, Rafael, Marco Aurélio Vaz, Aliaa Rehan Youssef, David Longino, and Walter Herzog. 2011."Changes in Contractile Properties of Muscles Receiving Repeat Injections of Botulinum Toxin (Botox)." *Journal of Biomechanics* 44, No. 1 : 39–44. https://doi.org/10.1016/j.jbiomech.2010.08.020.

Galatar, Adriana. 2021."7 Lucruri Pe Care Utilizatorii de Scaune Rulante Doresc Să Le Știi Despre Viața Lor Sexuală."Life in Progress. Last updated November 27, 2021. https://www.lifeinprogress.ro/7-lucruri-pe-care-utilizatorii-de-scaune-rulante-doresc-sa-le-stii-despre-viata-lor-sexuala/.

Goția, Dan, George, and Ardelean, Mircea. (1993). "Deviațiile axiale ale genunchiului". In *Elemente de chirurgie și ortopedie pediatrica*, 199-200. Iași, RO:Contact Internațional Atma S.R.L.

Goția, Dan, George, and Ardelean, Mircea. (1993). "Piciorul plat static". In *Elemente de chirurgie și ortopedie pediatrica*, 200-201. Iași, RO:Contact Internațional Atma S.R.L.

Goția, Dan, George, and Ardelean, Mircea. (1993). "Deformatiile degetelor". *In Elemente de chirurgie și ortopedie pediatrica*, 202.Iași, RO:Contact Internațional Atma S.R.L.

Graham, H.Kerr, K.Roger Aoki, Ilona Autti-Rämö, Roslyn N Boyd, Mauricio R Delgado, Deborah J Gaebler-Spira, Mark E Gormley, et al., 2000, "Recommendations for the Use of Botulinum Toxin Type A in the Management of Cerebral Palsy." *Gait & Posture* 11, No. 1: 67–79. https://doi.org/10.1016/s0966-6362(99)00054-5.

Graham, H. Kerr, Roslyn Boyd, John B Carlin, Fiona Dobson, Kevin Lowe, Gary Nattrass, Pam Thomason, Rory Wolfe, and Dinah Reddihough. 2008. "Does Botulinum Toxin a Combined with Bracing Prevent Hip Displacement in Children with Cerebral Palsy and 'Hips at Risk'*?" The Journal of Bone and Joint Surgery*, American Volume 90, No. 1: 23–33. https://doi.org/10.2106/jbjs.f.01416.

Graham, H.K. 2019. Unpublished data.

Greenough, W. T. and Chang, F. F. 1989. "Plasticity of synapse structure and pattern in the cerebral cortex". In A. Peters and E. G. Jones (Eds*.), Cerebral Cortex*, Vol. 7, 391–440. New York: Plenum Press.

Hartnett, M. Elizabeth, and Robert H. Lane. 2013. "Effects of Oxygen on the Development and Severity of Retinopathy of Prematurity." *Journal of American Association for Pediatric Ophthalmology and Strabismus* 17, No. 3: 229–34. https://doi.org/10.1016/j.jaapos.2012.12.155.

"Hemorzon Unguent, 18G, Antibiotice: Dr.Max Farmacie." Dr. Max Farmacie. Last updated December 15, 2022. https://www.drmax.ro/hemorzon-ung-18g-antibiotice.

Hoyto. "Clip-N-Pull: Pants Assist Dressing Aid." Last updated September 27, 2011. http://firstaidkitsdiscount.blogspot.com/2011/08/clip-n-pull-pants-assist-dressing-aid.html.

Jankovic, Joseph. 2004. "Botulinum Toxin in Clinical Practice" *Journal of Neurology, Neurosurgery & Psychiatry* 75, No. 7: 951–57. https://doi.org/10.1136/jnnp.2003.034702.

Johnston, R. B. 1976. ''Motor function: normal development and cerebral palsy". *In Developmental disorders: Assessment, treatment, education*, edited by Johnston R.B. and P. R. Magrab. Baltimore: University Park Press.

Karabay, Hasan, Müslüm Arıcı, and Murat Sandık. 2013."A Numerical Investigation of Fluid Flow and Heat Transfer inside a Room for Floor Heating and Wall Heating Systems." *Energy and Buildings* 67: 471–78. https://doi.org/10.1016/j.enbuild.2013.08.037.

Kaur, Amandeep. 2017. "Cerebral Palsy." Share and Discover Knowledge on SlideShare. Accessed May 28, 2023. https://www.slideshare.net/GAMANDEEP/cerebral-palsy-80482237.

Kelly, Evelyn B. 2013. *Encyclopedia of human genetics and disease*. Vol. 1. Santa Barbara, CA: Greenwood.

Khazaeni, Leila M. 2023."Strabismus - Children's Health Issues." MSD Manual Consumer Version. Last updated September, 2022. https://www.msdmanuals.com/home/children-s-health-issues/eye-disorders-in-children/strabismus.

Kolb, B., and Gibb, R. 2011. "Brain plasticity and behaviour in the developing brain". *Journal of the Canadian Academy of Child and Adolescent Psychiatry* 20, No.4: 265–276.

Kolb, Bryan, and Ian Q. Whishaw. 2015. "Neurodevelopmental disorders". In Fundamentals of Human Neuropsychology, 7th ed., 671–698. New York, NY: Worth Publishers.

Koman, L. Andrew, James F. Mooney, Beth Smith, Amy Goodman, and Theresa Mulvaney. 1993. "Management of Cerebral Palsy with Botulinum-A Toxin." *Journal of Pediatric Orthopaedics* 13, No. 4 : 489–95. https://doi.org/10.1097/01241398-199307000-00013.

Lebiedowska, Maria K., Siddhartha Sikdar, Avinash Eranki, and Lindsay Garmirian. "Knee Joint Angular Velocities and Accelerations during the Patellar Tendon Jerk. 2011." *Journal of Neuroscience Methods* 198, No. 2: 255–59. https://doi.org/10.1016/j.jneumeth.2011.04.018.

Lindemann J.E. 1981. "Cerebral Palsy". In*: Psychological and Behavioral Aspects of Physical Disability: A Manual for Health Practitioners* (1st ed.)(pp. 117-145). New York, NY: Plenum Press.

Linds Rehabilitation Equipment. n.d. "Ergo ReJoy, Active Controls Joystick." Linds Rehabilitation Equipment. Accessed May 30, 2023. https://www.lindsrehab.com.au/wheelchairs/wheelchair-accessories/ergo-rejoy-active-controls-joystick.html.

Little, William John. 1862 "On the Influence of Abnormal Parturition, Difficult Labours, Premature Birth and Asphyxia Neonatorum." Essay. *In*

Transactions of the Obstetrical Society of London 3, 3:293–344. London: Longman, Green, Longman, and Roberts.

Mandurah Physiotherapy. n.d. "Flat Feet vs High Foot Arch." Last updated January 19, 2018. Accessed May 18, 2023. https://www.mandurahphysiotherapy.com.au/high-foot-arch/.

Mendioroz Iriarte, M., and J.J. Poza. Aldea. 2003. "Mielopatía y Radiculopatía Por Cervicoartrosis. Tumores de La Médula Espinal." *Medicine - Programa de Formación Médica Continuada Acreditado* 8, No. 99: 5339–44. https://doi.org/10.1016/s0304-5412(03)70990-1.

Micheli, Federico E. 2002.*Tratado de neurología Clínica.* Buenos Aires: Editorial Médica Panamericana.

Minamoto, Viviane B., Kentaro P. Suzuki, Shannon N. Bremner, Richard L. Lieber, and Samuel R. Ward. 2015. "Dramatic Changes in Muscle Contractile and Structural Properties after 2 Botulinum Toxin Injections." *Muscle & Nerve* 52, No. 4: 649–57. https://doi.org/10.1002/mus.24576.

Minear, W. L. 1956. "Special Article: A classification of cerebral palsy" *Pediatrics* 18, No. 5: 841–52. https://doi.org/10.1542/peds.18.5.841.

Ministerie van Volksgezondheid, Welzijn en Sport .n.d. "Aankleedhulpmiddel Voor Broek of Rok". Accessed May 11, 2023. https://hulpmiddelenwijzer.nl/hulpmiddelen/aankleedhulpmiddelen-broek-rok.

Montastruc, Jeanne, Philippe Marque, Florence Moulis, Véronique Bourg, Valérie Lambert, Geneviève Durrieu, Jean-Louis Montastruc, and François Montastruc. 2016. "Adverse Drug Reactions of Botulinum Neurotoxin Type A in Children with Cerebral Palsy: A Pharmaco-Epidemiological Study in VigiBase." *Developmental Medicine & Child Neurology* 59, No. 3: 329–34. https://doi.org/10.1111/dmcn.13286.

Multani, Iqbal, Jamil Manji, Tandy Hastings-Ison, Abhay Khot, and Kerr Graham. 2019. "Botulinum Toxin in the Management of Children with Cerebral Palsy." *Pediatric Drugs* 21, No. 4: 261–81. https://doi.org/10.1007/s40272-019-00344-8.

Multani, Iqbal, Jamil Manji, Min Jia Tang, Walter Herzog, Jason J. Howard, and H. Kerr Graham. 2019. "Sarcopenia, Cerebral Palsy, and Botulinum Toxin Type A." *JBJS Reviews* 7, No. 8: 1–10. https://doi.org/10.2106/jbjs.rvw.18.00153.

Muscle and joint clinic. n.d. "Genu Valgum." Mississauga and Oakville Chiropractor and Physiotherapy Clinic - FREE Consult!, Last updated February 2, 2023. https://muscleandjoint.ca/genu-valgum/.

Nelson, K. B., and Ellenberg, J. H. 1978. Epidemiology of cerebral palsy. In B.S. Schoenberg, *Advances in Neurology,* 19, 421–435.

Neomed.ro. n.d. "Cadru de Mers Pliabil Cu 4 Roti Si Frana - RP742". Accessed May 11, 2023. https://neomed.ro/cadre-de-mers/1742-cadru-de-mers-pliabil-cu-4-roti-si-frana-rp742.html

Neurogen.in. n.d. "What Is Cerebral Palsy?" Cerebral Palsy - Cell Therapy. Accessed May 14, 2023. https://www.neurogen.in/cerebral-palsy

Nober, E.H. Auditory processing.1976. In W. M. Cruickshank (Ed.), *Cerebral palsy: A developmental disability*. Syracuse, N.Y.: Syracuse University Press.

Okazii. ro. n.d. "Talonete Magnetice Pentru Presopunctura." Okazii.ro. Accessed May 15, 2023. https://www.okazii.ro/talonete-magnetice-pentru-presopunctura-a192186509.

Orsini, Marco, Marco Antonio Araujo Leite, Tae Mo Chung, Wladimir Bocca, Jano Alves de Souza, Olivia Gameiro de Souza, Rayele Priscila Moreira, Victor Hugo Bastos, Silmar Teixeira, Acary Bulle Oliveira, Bruno da Silva Moraes, Matta André Palma, and Luis Jorge Jacinto. 2015. "Botulinum Neurotoxin Type A in Neurology: Update". *Neurology International* 7, No:2: 31-35.https://doi.org/10.4081/ni.2015.5886.

O'Sullivan, Rory, Damien Kiernan, Michael Walsh, Tim O'Brien, and Yahya Elhassan. 2016. "Characterisation of the Patellar Tendon Reflex in Cerebral Palsy Children Using Motion Analysis." *Irish Journal of Medical Science (1971 -)* 185, No. 4:813–17. https://doi.org/10.1007/s11845-015-1369-3.

Palmer M. L., Epler M. E. 2002. *Fundamentos de las Tecnicas de Evaluación Musculo Esqueletica* (Bicolor) 1st. Vol. 1. Badalona, Spain: Paidotribo.

Person. 2019. "VIDEO&FOTO: Multă Adrenalină Și Veselie În Parcul de Distracții Din Cicoarei." Ziarul de Iași - liderul presei iesene. Last updated October 12, 2019. https://www.ziaruldeiasi.ro/stiri/videofoto-multa-adrenalina-si-veselie-in-parcul-de-distractii-din-cicoarei--233047.html.

Piseru, Emanuel-Andrei, and Piseru Teodora. 2023. "Organizarea programului de terapie în pareză și plegie"(presentation, "Zilele Spitalului Clinic De Recuperare-Iași Conferinţa Națională „Paradigme În Recuperarea Medicală: De La Consens La Contradicţii,', Iași, 29 March, 1–14, edition 21.

Reiter and Walsh. n.d. "Gross Motor Function Classification System (GMFCS) for Cerebral Palsy." Last updated January 22, 2023. Accessed on 18 May, 2023. https://www.abclawcenters.com/cerebral-palsy/gross-motor-function-classification-system.

Ricard, François. 2003. *Tratamiento osteopático de las lumbalgias Y lumbociáticas por hernias discales. Madrid: Editorial Médica Panamericana.*

Sethu Child Development and Family Guidance. 2005. "Cerebral Palsy." Sethu. Accessed May 14, 2023. https://sethu.in/cerebral-palsy/.

Shumway-Cook, Anne, and Woollacott, Marjorie H. 2011. *Motor control - Translating research into clinical practice.*4th edition. Ed. Lippincott Williams & Wilkins.

Sirevaag, Anita M., and William T. Greenough. 1988."A Multivariate Statistical Summary of Synaptic Plasticity Measures in Rats Exposed to Complex, Social and Individual Environments." *Brain Research* 441, No. 1–2: 386–92. https://doi.org/10.1016/0006-8993(88)91420-5.

Smartiz.ro. n.d. "Talonete Ortopedice - Branturi CU Suport Platfus Arcul Piciorului." Smartiz.ro. Accessed May 15, 2023. https://www.smartiz.ro/produs/talonete-ortopedice-branturi-cu-suport-platfus-arcul-piciorului/

Smidt, Gary L, and Mark W Rogers. 1982. "Factors Contributing to the Regulation and Clinical Assessment of Muscular Strength." *Physical Therapy* 62, No. 9 : 1283–90. https://doi.org/10.1093/ptj/62.9.1283.

Stamatin, Maria, Păduraru, Luminița, and Avasiloaiei, Andreea-Luciana. 2009. *Neonatologie*. Iaşi: Editura "Gr. T. Popa", 57-60.

SunriseMedical. n.d. "Quickie Q7 Lightweight Rigid Wheelchair." Sunrise Medical. Accessed May 29, 2023.
https://www.sunrisemedical.com/manual-wheelchairs/quickie/rigid-wheelchairs/q7.

The Podiatry Institute. 2004. "TECHNIQUES OF GASTROCNEMIUS RECESSION". In *Update 2004: The Proceedings of the Annual Meeting of The Podiatry Institute.*

Tham, Lai Kuan, Noor Azuan Abu Osman, Wan Abu Wan Abas, and Kheng Seang Lim. 2013. "The Validity and Reliability of Motion Analysis in Patellar Tendon Reflex Assessment." *PLoS ONE* 8, No. 2: 1–6. e55702.
https://doi.org/10.1371/journal.pone.0055702.

Tortora, Gerard J., Bryan Derrickson, Karina Tzal, María de los Ángeles Gutiérrez, and Diana Klajn. 2002. *Principios de anatomía y fisiología*. Vol. 7. OXFORD University Press.

Tin, W, and S Gupta. 2007. "Optimum Oxygen Therapy in Preterm Babies." *ADC Fetal & Neonatal Edition*. https://doi.org/10.1136/adc.2005.092726.

Therapies for Kids. n.d."Treatment for Flat Feet." Therapies For Kids. Last updated May 18, 2023. Accessed May 19, 2023.
https://therapiesforkids.com.au/flat-feet/.

Turhan, Yalçın, and Mehmet Arıcan. 2019. "Clinical Comparison of Percutaneous and Open Hamstring Lengthening in Children with Spastic Cerebral Palsy." *Medeniyet Medical Journal*, 182-187 .
https://doi.org/10.5222/mmj.2019.54670.

Waterhouse, James, and Iain Campbell. 2008. "Reflexes: Principles and Properties." *Anaesthesia &Intensive Care Medicine* 9, No. 5: 210–15.
https://doi.org/10.1016/j.mpaic.2008.03.010.

Werner, David. 2011. *Where there is no doctor: A village health care handbook*. Palo Alto, CA.: Hesperian Foundation.

www.innobyte.ro, Innobyte Development -. "Cadru de Mers Fix, Reglabil" Rosal Ortopedic – Proteze, Orteze, Incaltaminte Ortopedica Si Dispozitive Pentru Mers." Rosal Ortopedic proteze orteze incaltaminte ortopedica si dispozitive pentru mers. Accessed May 11, 2023.
http://www.rosal-ortopedic.ro/produse/dispozitive-de-mers/cadru-de-mers/cadru-de-mers-fix-reglabil/.

Wikieducator.ro. n.d. "Lesson 20: Disability and Rehabilitation Part 2." WikiEducator. Accessed May 14, 2023.
https://wikieducator.org/Lesson_20:_Disability_and_Rehabilitation_Part_2.

YouTube."The Point of No Return | Tedy Necula | TEDxCambridgeSchoolofBucharest". Youtube video, 27:20. April 26, 2018.
https://www.youtube.com/watch?v=9X2KZy9x7WE.

Zorii, Andrii. 2019. "Children`s Developing Toy. the Labyrinth of Wooden Beads Isolated on White Baskground Stock Photo - Image of Line, Labyrinth: 164764178." Dreamstime. Last updated December 6, 2019.
https://www.dreamstime.com/children-s-developing-toy-labyrinth-wooden-beads-isolated-white-baskground-fine-motor-skills-image164764178.

LIST OF CONTRIBUTORS

Ioniță Brigitte
"Alexandru cel Bun" Secondary School, Iași, Romania

Păduraru Claudia-Andreea
Faculty of Visual Arts and Design George Enescu Iași, Romania

Piseru Emanuel-Andrei
Physiokinetotherapist specialist at Clinical Rehabilitation Hospital of Iași, Romania

Vieriu Iuliana-Ilinca
Faculty of Visual Arts and Design George Enescu Iași, Romania

INDEX